It's
Not
ABOUT
the
Food

It's Not ABOUT the Food

Mary Perry

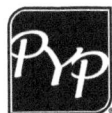

PUBLISH YOUR PURPOSE PRESS

Publish Your Purpose Press
141 Weston Street, #155
Hartford, CT, 06141

PUBLISH
YOUR
PURPOSE
PRESS

The opinions expressed by the Author are not necessarily those held by Publish Your Purpose Press.

Ordering Information: Quantity sales and special discounts are available on quantity purchases by corporations, associations, and others. For details, contact the publisher at orders@publishyourpurposepress.com.

Edited by: Erin Walton, Heidi King, and Wendie Pecharsky
Cover design by: Cornelia Murariu
Typeset by: Medlar Publishing Solutions Pvt Ltd., India

Printed in the United States of America.
ISBN: 978-1-951591-57-1 (paperback)
ISBN: 978-1-951591-58-8 (ebook)

Library of Congress Control Number: 2021900582

First edition, February 2021

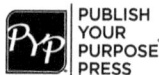

The mission of Publish Your Purpose Press is to discover and publish authors who are striving to make a difference in the world. We give marginalized voices power and a stage to share their stories, speak their truth, and impact their communities. Do you have a book idea you would like us to consider publishing? Please visit PublishYourPurposePress.com for more information.

TABLE OF CONTENTS

CHAPTER 1

INTRODUCTION: SINGLE STEP

*The journey of a thousand miles
begins with a single step.*
— Lao Tzu, ancient Chinese philosopher

I have loved this quote of Lao Tzu since I was a young child. A poster of it hung on the wood-paneled walls of our finished basement: "The journey of a thousand miles begins with a single step." Under the letters, a tiny, fuzzy, yellow duckling with sweet, innocent black eyes waddled out of a large wooden barrel tipped on its side. The precious bundle of feathers was making its way into a large field, and the contrast between the sunshine yellow of its fur against the backdrop of tall vibrant-green grass mesmerized me. I used to sit on the orange carpet in front of that poster, lean back with my arms propped behind me, considering the words and picture. At the time, the world seemed like such an overwhelming place, and I took comfort in that innocent, fragile duckling stepping forward into the unknown. If that small creature could be so brave, so could I.

I know that many of my clients, when they take that first step through my door, may be experiencing those same mixed fuzzy-yellow-duckling-poster feelings—nervous, excited, overwhelmed . . . and also hopeful. They often have dieted for many years and lost the same weight over and over again. They are skeptical that they will be successful working with someone new since they have been trying for what feels like their whole lives to lose weight and keep it off. Often, they have engaged in restrictive diets that forbid certain foods with the promise that *this* is finally the lasting answer—their problems will be solved once and for all.

But nothing works, and they find themselves ensnared in a pattern of feeling insecure, out of control, and uncertain how to find positive and lasting change. Feeling defeated, they often turn to food for comfort, getting stuck in a cycle of overeating and then restricting. They think if they can find the right plan, all will be OK.

What they don't understand is that it's not about the food at all. They will soon realize, just as I did, that their issues have very little to do with food.

The first question I always ask a new client is: "Why did you come to see me today?" While they may say it's to lose weight or improve their bloodwork, they always start by telling me their story.

DEE'S STORY

Dee,* a single mother in her early 40s, is successful in her career as a social worker but has always struggled with her weight. Having dieted for most of her life, she has lost the same 40–50 pounds over and over again. Growing up, she watched her mom struggle under the double burden of excess weight and her dad's degrading comments about her appearance. Her dad also got mad if he didn't get the last bites of food in the chip bag or ice cream container. Dee and her mom would wait until he went to bed so they could stay up late watching TV and sneaking junk food.

Now as an adult, Dee struggles with a desire to eat mostly snack food instead of meals and gets extremely sad or upset if she

---

*All client names have been changed to protect their privacy.

can't eat what she wants. She has two young kids and puts their needs first, including making them healthy meals, but she will then snack on junk food herself. She feels exhausted and stressed most of the time, and the thought of trying to eat healthy food and lose weight is overwhelming. At the same time, however, she's worried about getting diabetes and not being able to take care of her family. She knows she should eat better and exercise, but she's been down this road before, and she's skeptical that she will ever be able to find a better path.

For people like Dee, just taking the first step and making an appointment can be extremely difficult. Many of my clients are women with established careers and family. They are often successful in many aspects of their personal and professional life but have had a lifelong struggle with food and managing their weight. Their relationship with food is the one area they haven't been able to make peace with, and they aren't sure what to expect when they come to see a dietitian. They worry it might be like visiting the food police, where someone will be judging them for their choices and handcuffing them with strict rules about what to eat and what not to eat. They often fear they will be judged in the same way they secretly have been judging themselves and that the visit will confirm their worst fears—that they are weak and a failure.

That is a far cry, however, from how I view these clients. The people who come to see me are some of the strongest people I know. They are the go-to people—the ones their family and friends always rely on. They are the caretakers who put everyone else's needs above their own, and they are used to being in this role. They tend to find validation of their worth by focusing on other people's needs and often have become so accustomed to being in this role that they find it terrifying to shift their focus onto themselves and then risk failure of not getting what they want. They may unconsciously feel unworthy of love and compelled to take care of others in order to earn love.

These clients begin to emotionally rely on food to meet their needs. Food becomes one of the few acceptable ways they treat themselves, and the thought of making changes to one of the few things that seems to bring safety, love, comfort, and a sense of importance feels scary. I understand this struggle because, as you will read in later chapters, this was me as well.

After years of relating to food in this way, some people realize the relationship has come at a price. They wake up to the fact that they have been sacrificing themselves and that their bondage to food has brought them to a place where they are not happy with their bodies and how they feel.

That's when they show up to see me.

My clients will often tell me, "I know what to do, but I'm just not doing it." Since they are usually the one fixing everything in their lives and attending to other's needs, they often feel they should have the solution. *After all*, they reason to themselves, *why do I need someone to tell me what I already know?* Since they are strong people, they feel they should be able to fix themselves, too.

But the truth in these situations is just the opposite. As one of my clients insightfully stated, "Strong people need support, too." I couldn't agree more. My role is to be your coach, your greatest supporter, and your facilitator of health and wellness. My job is to help guide you as we work together as a team to create a new path that bridges the gap between your habits and lifestyle now and where you want to go. The thing I love about my work is that I'm there *just for you*. Nobody else. When you're so used to being the one taking care of everyone else, having someone care about just what *you* need is, I think, a crucial piece of the puzzle. The helpers need help, too.

Dee needed help to discover that her struggles with eating and managing her weight were not really about the food. They were about how her past history and learned coping mechanisms were playing into her current lifestyle and creating a dysfunctional relationship with food by relying on it as the main tool to manage her emotional needs.

Dee and I worked together on meal planning to create quick, healthy, and enjoyable meals that were both physically and emotionally satisfying. We also identified ways to feel relaxed and emotionally nourished that didn't involve snack food. This was a key component for Dee in achieving a healthier relationship with food.

Other practices Dee began incorporating in her life included:

- pausing before automatically reaching for chips or ice cream. This gave her time to consider her choices and reflect on whether she was craving food due to physical hunger or emotional reasons.
- knowing that no foods were off-limits and that she always had permission to eat what she wanted. This changed her mindset from one of restriction to one of empowerment fostered by actively making choices about what to eat.
- finding ways to take care of herself the way she took care of her kids in order to help put herself higher on her priority list.

Dee continues to have a healthier relationship with food by practicing the strategies we worked on. She has found a balance of enjoying food while nourishing herself without needing to rely on overwhelming portions to manage her feelings. She sometimes eats a food because it's comforting, but she is able to choose a portion that feels satisfying and manageable by tuning into what she is eating while she fully enjoys and embraces the experience.

ELLA'S STORY

Ella was another client who came to see me to get help with losing weight. She told me she was balancing a full-time job while taking care of her family and her mom. Every day she would visit her mom after work and cook her meals, do household chores, and help her bathe so her mom could live independently in her home. Ella would often take time off from work to bring her mother to medical appointments. Because her mom needed to gain weight, she would cook familiar Southern meals from her childhood that included fried foods and side dishes with generous amounts of butter. She would also buy fast food to entice her mom to eat. She felt exhausted from doing so much and struggled to lose weight as she ate large portions of the high-calorie foods she made or bought for her mom out of convenience.

Ella's core issue in managing her weight was not about the food but about how to care for herself in the midst of juggling all her responsibilities and taking care of everyone else's needs. She was putting herself last on the list, which led to neglecting the food and movement choices she needed to support her health.

Ella and I worked together to identify and practice incorporating nutrition and wellness strategies that allowed her to balance caring for herself while also caring for others. The first step was modifying what she was cooking for her mom so she would have healthier meals to eat herself while still providing foods that would serve her mother's needs. We also identified healthier fast-food options she could order from restaurants when she was bringing food home for her mom. And we strategized about having other family members participate in her mom's care so Ella could have time for daily, stress-relieving movement, such as walking or yoga.

For so many clients, on the surface of their lives, food seems to be the issue, but it's actually not about the food at all. It's not about eating fewer sweets. It's about a client's daughter unexpectedly passing away and candy and cookies becoming the only thing that provided enough of a distraction to make existing barely tolerable. It's not about the fast food; it's about the client whose spouse took his own life and just the thought of sitting down and eating a balanced meal without him being too painful.

These stories are just two of the many examples in my experience that stand out to me because they are representative of the struggle that many of my clients face with their health and weight when food is used as the main tool to manage their emotions, feelings, and stress or when they neglect themselves and their nutritional needs in their caretaking roles.

YOUR STORY

Everyone has a story. I believe that your story matters, too.

This book/guide is not about what to eat, low carb versus high carb, or the most magical diet. It's about examining what food *means to you*; identifying how your mindset, thoughts, and emotions impact your choices and learning through small steps how to heal those parts of yourself in order to transform your relationship with food.

My goal is to help you identify and analyze the root causes of what is driving your behavior and to give you strategies that allow you to retrain your mindset. Creating a fresh mental map constructs a new pathway that allows different habits to form, helping you to meet your goals in the long term and to freely live your best life.

In the following chapters, you will learn:

- how to include foods you love to eat and still meet your health and weight goals;
- strategies for getting "unstuck" by having a process to implement incremental daily healthy habits;
- techniques to become aware of the reasons you eat and to learn how to insert pauses between thinking and acting so you can fully embrace your choices;
- how small changes can add up to life-changing results.

This book is a compilation of my own transformational experiences as I healed my relationship with food, as well as the insights I've gained from many years as a dietitian coaching thousands of clients. The pages of this book drove me to write them because I, too, know the suffering that weighs a person down when eating feels overwhelming and unmanageable, causing one to become stuck in a body, mindset, and pattern that leads to hopelessness and misery.

My purpose is to help others who are struggling with their relationship with food and to let you know you are not alone. Many other people are struggling with the same issues. In this book, I identify the key mental and emotional changes I've experienced, witnessed, and supported in many clients that must accompany nutritional changes in order to make a transformational difference. It's the difference between being successful in liberating yourself or staying stuck in destructive patterns.

I've gathered all these lessons learned to provide strategies to help you get started and support you along the way. As we take this journey together, my goal is to help you feel hopeful again by believing that you will be successful because you now have specific steps to start changing your thinking and behavior. You can now begin making changes by taking small steps, no matter where you are in your journey.

Now, more than ever, we need to practice kindness, love, and compassion—especially to ourselves—in every area of our lives. Change is always challenging, but that doesn't mean we have to do it alone. I'm here to help and guide you along the way.

Before we continue, I want to thank you for taking this journey with me. This book is a love letter to myself to honor and acknowledge my journey, to all my clients who have trusted in me to help guide them on their journey, and to you, my readers, who have the faith to read this book and be open to a new way of looking at your relationship with food. Even though we haven't met in person yet, I am honored to work with you through this medium. I am always humbled and very appreciative when my clients share their story with me and let me into their lives. Thank you for letting me into yours.

To begin, I would like to let you into my life by sharing some of my story with you.

CHAPTER 2

MY STORY: WHY IT WASN'T ABOUT THE FOOD FOR ME

*Tell your story because your story will heal you
and it will heal someone else.*
— Iyanla Vanzant

Growing up, I loved food. Food was delicious and fun and comforting, but I often felt like food didn't love me back. It betrayed me by giving me a body that was often told it was flawed. My relationship with food was as confusing as when a childhood crush is mean to you and a grown-up responds, "It's because they like you." Huh? It made no sense to me, and I struggled with a love-hate relationship with food for many years.

In my early years, images of TV-defined beauty fascinated me. They offered both hope and struggle as I tried to reconcile how I looked with what I saw. Figuring out how to eat to transform myself into the images on TV felt like a Rubik's Cube puzzle I could never solve. To make things more confusing, I often used food as my emotional Band-Aid, which made it difficult to distinguish between physical and emotional hunger.

Standing in front of the freezer, eating ice cream candy bars until I felt sick was how I tried to stuff down feelings of depression at home during the summer after my freshman year of college.

When I returned to college, continuing unhappiness sent me to the vending machines late at night, where I could choose a variety of junk food to eat in secret. I felt I deserved treats when I gave too much of myself and no one else seemed to care about my needs. Bingeing on pizza and large Heath Bar Crunch cookies made me feel special and soothed the pain.

Food became a way to manage feelings of unworthiness, depression, unhappiness, and loneliness that I couldn't articulate at the time. Eating became a vehicle to prove that I mattered, I was special, and I deserved to be treated as such.

Sometimes clients will believe that because my body is a certain size, I haven't grappled with weight issues. I usually share that I struggled for many years. The difficulties and challenges I experienced served a purpose that was only revealed later on—my journey to heal myself ignited the desire to return to school to become a dietitian. I wanted to merge educational expertise with what I had learned personally so I could help others in pain and struggling with similar issues. I hate to see others suffering, and my passion and purpose is to do anything I can to help alleviate such pain.

Even though I was always the "heavy" one in the family, I didn't initially realize I was overweight or that I needed to change anything. I was a pretty happy kid until people started pointing out my weight to me. One of my earliest memories of this is being at the pediatrician's office for my annual physical when I was maybe around six or seven years old. For starters, as the doctor's pokes and prods tickled me, he met my smiles, laughter, and squirms with sober reserve. When the exam was complete, I hopped off the examination table and stood in the small, dark-wood-paneled room between my mother and the doctor. I felt like a short invisible net between two badminton players as their conversation shuttlecock flew back and forth over my head before landing heavily on the court: "She's a good 15 pounds overweight and needs to lose weight," the doctor stated dryly. *Hello, I'm standing right here; I can hear you,* my mind protested silently. Somehow the doctor hadn't thought it was important to include me in the conversation or even acknowledge my existence, except for the fact that my body needed to change.

Reflecting on this now makes me realize this was one of the earliest memories that planted the seed of belief that I was not good enough or worthy because of how I looked.

Do you have a moment like this that stands out in your mind? Do you have any memories of someone or something causing you to look at your body in a negative light? Is this still affecting how you see yourself today?

Another memory took place a few years later in music class as I joined my classmates seated in lines on cold, metal folding chairs. While we waited for the class to start singing, a boy in elementary school strode up to me in anger, taunting, "Why are you fat when no one else in your family is? I'm going to punch you in the face at recess because you're fat!" I just stared at him with large deer eyes, not sure how to respond to avoid harm, praying I would magically be unseen. The feeling of being hated for how I looked still lingers today. It left the impression that I was at fault for making him so angry and that it was my responsibility to change myself to be protected.

Around this time, I started taking swimming lessons. After I completed the eight-week course, someone innocently noted, "Wow, you've really slimmed down." Their comment puzzled me; I was shrinking, taking up less space, and being applauded for it. My brain became indoctrinated early: fat "bad"—you get punched in the face, skinny or slim "good"—you get praised. Having grown up attending a small private Catholic school, I understood rules, and I figured out that all I had to do was follow this new one to succeed and feel worthy. My young brain interpreted the "rules" to mean that I had to learn to manipulate food to transform my body into someone who could be loved.

Do you have any instances where you felt you needed to be a certain size or shape to be accepted or to accept yourself? My story may be reminding you of things that have happened in your life as well. Think about how you viewed your body; did that view impact your relationship with food? Did it make you change your food choices or how much you ate? Like my experiences did for me, did yours create a love-hate relationship between eating and your body?

TV: THE ORIGINAL ESCAPE ROUTE

My feelings of not being good enough and not deserving of love unless I looked a certain way shaped me (pun intended) in many ways. As a young girl, I watched sanitized and romanticized versions of life on TV. I loved shows such as *The Love Boat, Fantasy Island, Dallas,* and *Charlie's Angels* along with *Happy Days, Laverne and Shirley,* and *Eight Is Enough.*

The *Love Boat* was a favorite, triggering fantasies of an adult life that somehow involved cruising to romantic places like Acapulco and Puerto Vallarta, Mexico. In my visions, I would be wearing bikinis with high heels along with sparkling jewelry and beaded evening gowns under long, voluminous hair, all while basking in the thrill of romantic escapades with my impossibly handsome husband. It makes me laugh to think back on this now—what a far cry from current-style staples of a ponytail and daily athleisure leggings and sneakers.

In one episode, a popular actress who was guest starring as "Wendy"—a woman on her honeymoon—would only let her new husband see her glamorous image. Julie, the cruise director, somehow realizes that Wendy is hiding a "dark secret" and goes to the woman's room. She stands there stunned as Wendy starts molting and peeling off the layers of her glamorous cover, throwing her Texas-large wig, fake lashes, foam breast inserts, and Lee Press On nails throughout the cabin, revealing her "plain," flat-chested true self. Under Julie's urging, Wendy shows up at breakfast as the real her and, in a ridiculous plot twist, her husband doesn't even recognize her. Ouch! But it's TV-land, so the husband comes around and loves his wife just for how she really looks, which of course, is still gorgeous and thin, just with fewer beauty accoutrements.

The message was that even though Wendy wasn't as physically beautiful as originally portrayed, her husband was still able to love her. The fact that she had to "trick" him to land him in the first place, however, reinforced the idea that our authentic selves aren't good enough.

This storyline resonated with me as I was a chubby kid with a Dorothy Hamill bowl haircut. It made such an impression that I still remember it so many years later. Wendy could get away with being less glamorous and still be loved by her husband because she remained so petite. In my mind, that meant that being thin ranked higher on the beauty scale than sporting fluffy hair and long eyelashes. *I may be ugly now*, I thought to myself, *but the future holds promise and possibility if I can change my body.*

There was hope. I dreamed that adulthood would give me the time and opportunity to transform myself into someone as beautiful, glamorous, and thin as the actresses on these shows— someone who deserved to be loved. It was not about the food. It was about using food to try and alter myself to become the vision I saw on TV.

Did you love any TV shows that affected how you saw yourself? Did the shows make you see yourself in a positive or negative light? Did you change your relationship with food because of how you saw yourself?

THE CHARO LESSON

Another reason I loved *The Love Boat* was that I would often visit my grandmother, and the two of us would sit and watch the show on Saturday nights. A frequent guest star on the show was Spanish-born actress, singer, musician, and all-around entertainer Charo. I loved Charo because she was everything I was not—talented, blonde, sexy, and sassy. Her catchphrase, "Cuchi-cuchi," uttered in unison with a wiggle of her hips, highlighted her bombshell looks and bubbly personality. When I expressed to my grandmother my undying affection for Charo, I was taken aback when she (gasp) said she didn't like Charo. Struggling to comprehend something so inconceivable, I asked her why. "Because Charo is not the type of girl to go to a party and sit quietly in the corner," my grandmother replied. "She needs to be the center of attention. Don't be like Charo."

That phrase—don't be like Charo—seeped into my subconscious mind like Kool-Aid soaked up by a Bounty paper towel. The message was, be yourself but not too much, and do it quietly. *Shrink yourself, shrink your body, be small.*

Most of the power of this message has dried out, but the sticky remnants remain crusted on my soul. I can see now how the idea of having to manipulate my personality and body to make it acceptable and pleasing to others played into my relationship with food. Instead of listening to myself and allowing my authenticity to shine through, I started making choices based on what I thought I should do instead of what I really wanted. Rather than eating the cupcake I craved, I chose the lettuce I didn't want.

My existence began to revolve around denial and deprivation instead of growth and fulfillment. I rebelled against this constriction by trying to control the only thing that seemed within my power—food. As I grew older, I realized that cupcakes and cookies were never going to satisfy my true need to be seen and heard. Overeating only temporarily quieted the mind, and when that moment had passed, more unhappiness followed.

Do you remember a time when someone tried to make you feel small or that you shouldn't be so "extra?" Did it make you want to change yourself physically? How did your feelings of self-worth affect your relationship with food then and now?

SWEET SMORGASBORD

My young concerns about appearance and body issues competed with the allure of food, especially sweets. I always loved parties as a kid because they were a socially acceptable chance to eat sweets. A lot of them! Catholic grade school holiday parties were the best because everyone would bring in homemade baked goods and candy. Oh, the *joy* of seeing my desk covered in brightly decorated cupcakes, cookies, and candy of all kinds.

Valentine's Day was a particular standout as the cupcakes and cookies were heart-shaped with the word *love* written in icing. Classmates deposited small, store-bought Valentines in brown paper bags taped to the front of our desks. Eating sweets while reading messages of love (even if you knew your classmates were forced to give everyone a Valentine) was comforting. With love displayed openly on my desk and the shame of indulging in a buffet of sweets nonexistent at that moment, I was temporarily free. Every year, Valentine's Day turned my desk into a safe space where I could eat what I wanted without feeling judged. I could be just another kid eating a cupcake instead of a kid who didn't deserve to enjoy treats because I was fat.

My favorite Valentine's Day treats were thick chocolate chip cookies made by a classmate's mom, with real butter! Although I did a lot of baking in those early years, I used margarine, which always made the cookies spread out flat and end up looking kind of sad and lifeless. Lisa's mom's cookies were dense, yet soft and perfectly shaped with large chocolate chips or, sometimes, even fancier white chocolate chips. Lisa's mom was not only a good baker but also what I considered glamorous; she was petite with a stylish brown bob haircut that always seemed to be perfectly in place. It amazed me how she could bake such delicious cookies and still be so beautiful and trim. Finding a peaceful balance between the urge to eat sweets and achieving the body I wanted felt like a magician's trick that I couldn't understand, and I feared I might never have the ability to master.

THE SHAMING JAMIE

The freedom of school parties always sent me sailing sky high because I never ordered dessert when eating out. My two skinny sisters always did, but I was too embarrassed by my fat body and felt I didn't deserve the sweet food. This decision seemed like a wise choice after a scarring episode one summer at a dinner with the family of a salesman who worked for my father. Their pre-teen daughter, Jamie, insisted on cutting me a piece of cake as large as a dinner plate and then presented it to me, as if announcing from the grandstands: "I know you can eat this because you're fat!" Jamie's dad gave her a disapproving look for a second while stating her name in reprimand, but other than that, the adults kept the conversation going. I sheepishly accepted the cake when Jamie refused to back down. After taking a few bites, I quietly said I didn't want it.

Have you ever experienced someone trying to shame you for eating or not eating something because of the size or shape of your body? How did you react? Did you try to shrink away quietly like I did, or did you stand up for yourself? Are your feelings about this still part of your story today?

LOVE WRAPPED IN FUR

Animals have always been a big source of comfort for me, especially dogs. Dogs are love wrapped in fur. They are nonjudgmental, affectionate, don't care what you look like, and just want to be with you. People can be very hard on other people, especially when it comes to appearance. Animals provide that quiet love and acceptance that shows us how we deserve to be treated by others as well as by ourselves, especially when we're struggling with self-image.

When I was around six years old, I visited my maternal grandmother at her cottage on a lake in Upstate New York after my grandfather passed away. The two-story wooden cottage had been built by my grandfather on a steep, tree-lined hill overlooking Canandaigua Lake. One of the most special things about that trip was walking down the dirt road to visit the two neighboring cottages. The summer homes were owned by two brothers who came to spend time there with their families. They collectively owned about five to six black Labs at any given time. As I made my way to their houses, a sea of black Labs would engulf me, and I would be submerged in hot fur, sloppy kisses, and pure joy. My favorite was an older dog named Gypsy. I would spend hours with her on the front porch, petting her in total bliss.

As a young child, I begged my family to get our own dog. After my father finally agreed to a pet, a classified ad in our local newspaper showed us our next step: "Free dog" it advertised. We drove out to a country farm in our blue station wagon with the windows down on a hot summer day. A pregnant dog that had been dropped off in the country had wandered to the farm and given birth there to her puppies. The farmer, clearly not interested in having any more animals on the property, was happy to offload the creatures as quickly as possible. I begged my mother for one of the puppies, but she agreed to take the mother dog instead. I was more than OK with that. The ride home was pure happiness, as our new dog, Clementine, slept on my lap in the back of the station wagon. Years later, my mother would recount the story and tell how she was afraid I would catch a disease from the dirty and sickly looking dog. I don't remember Clementine like that at all. To me, she was always beautiful.

One summer when I was 11 or 12, my sister, her friend, and I were bored, so we decided to put together a Hawaiian-themed dinner for our two families. Excitement filled the air as everyone got into the spirit and dressed up in grass skirts and leis. I happily sported a new outfit of white shorts and a blue, short-sleeved polo shirt with rainbow stripes across the chest. A flower in my hair and a grass skirt finished off the look. Because I was overweight, however, the grass skirt wrapped only part way around me, leaving at least a five- or six-inch gap where the ends of the skirt should have met. Some of the family members pointed out the gap and laughed quietly at me. A picture taken that night shows me with the families in the backyard, smiling but clutching my friend's miniature black poodle, Monique, to my chest, with my face resting on hers.

In difficult moments like these, dogs always showed me it was not about the food and how it made me look; it was about being loved. I loved dogs, and, unlike food, they loved me back. Unconditionally. Their acceptance was a constant, so different from the relationship I had with food. In the presence of others, I often felt that food was conditional and had to be earned. In the quiet moments by myself, however, food felt just the opposite; the soft, sweet, gooey, iced Honey Bun snack cake always seemed to accept me for who I was as it beckoned me to eat and feel happy.

Did you have someone or something that made you feel totally accepted, especially when not feeling positive about yourself? Do you still have that in your life now? Is there a food that seems to speak to you and make you feel comforted and cared for? Are you able to enjoy it now without having to eat an amount that feels overwhelming? If not, what is the food giving you that you are not getting from yourself or others?

AVOIDING THE FRESHMAN 15

The first time I tried to lose weight, I was in high school. (I'll tell you more about my struggles during this time in a later chapter.)

When I went to college, my focus on weight loss continued. During my freshman year there, I started skipping lunch and drinking just a SlimFast shake for breakfast and a salad for dinner. Determined to avoid the dreaded "Freshman 15" weight gain, I began walking obsessively for one hour daily, then two hours or more. By the end of the year, I couldn't keep this regimen up and started eating. The strict deprivation led to binge eating and feeling out of control. The thrill of having been congratulated for losing weight during high school and achieving a certain body dissolved into extreme shame, and I continued binge eating over the next few years as I gained 40–45 pounds.

As I was getting ready to graduate from college and looking for interview outfits, I realized I couldn't fit into any clothes in the store. My "why" for change became crystal clear—I was making choices that weren't honoring me, how I wanted to feel, or who I wanted to be, and I was carrying this unhappiness on my body. That day was a turning point, as I saw myself at a crossroads: I could keep doing what I was doing and become more enmeshed in a cycle of restricting and bingeing or I could take a different path.

I struggled with binge eating episodes for several years after that, but I worked hard to dissolve the strong tie to emotional eating and put food in its place. I deciphered the magician's trick of finding peace with my body and the role of food in my life. My struggle to live a healthier life inspired me to return to school in my early 30s and become a dietitian. I suffered a lot for many years, and my desire to help others so they wouldn't have to suffer like I did ignited a passion that has only grown more intense, even after 12 years as a dietitian.

I'm a pretty private person, but I feel it's important to share my story because people often assume I haven't dealt with difficulty in the area of food because of how I look now. However, I know the struggle well. Yes, it was a long road, but I have come out on the other side—stronger and healthier. The purpose of this book is to help you do the same.

CHAPTER 3

THE ROLE OF FOOD

Food brings people together on many different levels.
It's nourishment of the soul and body; it's truly love.
— Giada De Laurentiis

As we started to explore in the previous chapter, you may be reflecting on the reasons you feel your relationship with food is such a continuous struggle. You want to lose weight, but you keep finding yourself overeating and making choices that don't support your goals. Why the constant push-pull? You try to push away what you deem unhealthy foods and large portions, but you keep getting sucked back into a never-ending food tornado. This vortex exists because food is much more than a functional way to fuel our bodies. Food provides love and comfort by the way it connects us to people, places, and memories and fills our physical and emotional needs.

I started to look at food differently when I first went to China six years ago. I was a late bloomer and hadn't done any significant international travel until after I turned 40. It was my first big trip outside the United States, and I was both excited and intimidated. I was traveling to Beijing as part of an international group to participate in an Olympic weightlifting camp. My adult fitness hobby had connected me with Olympic weightlifting, and I jumped at the chance to attend a camp where we were to stay in the dorms at Beijing Sport University and train twice a day with the team there.

Meals were a big part of that experience. We ate breakfast and lunch buffet style on campus but patronized local restaurants for dinner. The restaurant meals were always served family style at large round tables that seated at least 15–20 people. Massive lazy Susans covered most of each table. The large, spinning platters held a variety of dishes filled with entrees such as steamed pork buns, Mapo tofu with spicy red sauce, flounder in black bean sauce, shredded beef or pork with green peppers, and green beans stir-fried with garlic and ginger. Tea flowed constantly, and the meals often ended with fresh watermelon.

Sharing these authentic meals family style in a foreign country with a group of people I had only recently met enhanced the weightlifting camp experience. It was not just about the food during the trip; it was about the uniqueness of the whole experience and the way we ate together that reinforced our sense of community in a new culture. Calories and fat and carbs were not concerns. I learned there that my main desire was for connection.

Food has a powerful ability to transport us back to a moment in time. In these memories, we find often comfort and happiness. One time when a niece came to visit, I let her eat chocolate ice cream with cookie dough—her favorite—for breakfast. It was a special treat, and I wanted her to experience the pure joy of eating something just for fun at a time she wouldn't normally indulge herself. It remains a special memory for me even though I wasn't the one eating the ice cream.

Food is also the way you connect with yourself. On a base level, you need food to live, but you have probably questioned why your mind and your physical hunger have become so disconnected. Consider how you have been conditioned to the positive and negative meanings of food as you, like most people, have experienced food being used for celebrations and rewards and love and caring as well as obligation and punishment.

For example, you may have bought cookies to thank people for helping you or chocolate to soothe your friend after they experienced a breakup. Maybe you grew up being rewarded with ice cream if you got good grades or punished with no dessert if you didn't clean your plate at dinner.

These push-pull messages—if you're "good" or "hurting," you get treats; if you're "bad," food gets withheld—start to turn food into a moral argument and a control issue rather than just food. Yet even when you "earn" your treat, you might still be deprived of or shamed for receiving it based on how you look. Eating becomes a very complicated sport, entangling you with sticky, spider-web-like rules.

Think about where and when food may have started to take on a darker meaning in your life. We all have those stories. One client shared with me how her father always laid claim to the last bite of food, whether from the chip bag or container of ice cream. If someone else polished it off first, he would become infuriated. Now, as an adult with freedom to buy and eat all the food she wanted, the client was struggling with dieting and the idea of any kind of food restriction. Another client and her cousin would buy snack food at the convenience store and then throw it through an open bathroom window at home, crawl in, and hide the food in the hamper. Later they would sneak in and secretly eat the hidden treasure because their mothers, who were attempting to control their children's weight, wouldn't allow such treats.

Food can become a compulsion or addiction if you grow up being restricted and getting messages that you don't deserve to nourish yourself. You learn that you have to sneak food in order to meet your physical needs. This causes a psychological toll, as later on in life, food takes on the role of soothing the emotional needs that weren't met during childhood. Overeating can become the norm as you stuff yourself with food to provide comfort, entertainment, or distraction. This is not weakness. This is trying to heal yourself in the only way you know how.

Occasionally eating for comfort or to soothe yourself is a natural and healthy part of balanced eating. We often eat chicken soup when feeling sick, drink a cup of cocoa on a snowy day, or eat breakfast for a Sunday-night dinner like when we were kids in order to feel both physically and psychologically nourished. Constantly using food as your main coping mechanism when you aren't being heard or emotionally getting what you need, however, causes other issues. You might find yourself in a body you're not comfortable in, experiencing a health issue for which you have to take medication, and/or feeling low energy or depressed, wondering how you got to this point.

People often judge the size and shape of another person's body as a reflection of that person's strength, character, self-control, work ethic, or willpower. I take a different view. I believe weight tells the story of your life. I want you to view your life through this lens as well. How you eat, what you eat, and how much you eat can provide clues as to what issues you're really dealing with. Becoming aware of the reasons you eat and learning how to put pauses between thinking and acting on your urges to eat will give you the time to thoughtfully consider your options so that you can fully embrace your choices. This will help you learn how to include the foods you love to eat in a balanced way that assists you in meeting your health goals. This is how you start to transform your relationship with food and change your life for its duration.

CHAPTER 4

MARTHA MARTYR AND THE EMOTIONAL BATH FITTER

When you say "yes" to others, make sure
you are not saying "no" to yourself.
— Paulo Coelho

It was a sticky summer afternoon, and I was riding with my two best friends, Jean and Mary Ellen, in a powder-blue station wagon, being chauffeured by Jean's mom. It was around 1980, a time when cars weren't automatically equipped with air conditioners unless you were "rich" and wanted to pay extra. I was laughing and smiling as the sun beat through the hot air of the open car windows, causing us to stick to the matching powder-blue pleather seats. I thought this was the coolest station wagon since it had rear-facing seats that allowed the occupants to wave or make faces at the cars following behind.

Even at a young age, Jean was the Queen Bee of the class. Her father was a doctor, which, in our small school, helped to elevate her to the top of the pecking order. She had long, blonde hair and wore glasses that only seemed to highlight her charming and outgoing personality. She was fun to be around and popular with the teachers and students alike. When she payed attention to you,

you felt special and accepted, too, because you became part of her golden circle.

At our first stop, we dropped Mary Ellen off at her home. Mary Ellen was petite, sweet, and agreeable—an ideal companion for Jean, who liked to be the center of attention. As she stepped out of the vehicle, Mary Ellen turned to Jean and asked, "What time are you arriving for the sleepover tonight?" "Around 7 p.m.," Jean replied.

The smile beginning on my face vanished almost as soon as it started as I realized I wasn't being included. Disappointment melted over me like a scoop of ice cream sliding off its cracked sugar cone base onto a sizzling sidewalk. Something once so sweet had been transformed into a sticky, lifeless puddle that people carefully avoided—a has-been who nobody wanted any longer. At that moment, even though I was invisible to my friends, I wanted to curl up and disappear from the whole world.

Though this interaction was painful, it should not have been a total surprise to me since a year or two earlier, when the three of us were on the playground together, my friends had turned to me and said, "We like each other a little bit more than we like you." I took in this shocking information with saucer eyes. "That's OK," I said. As a kid, I thought that being nice meant being accepting and understanding and not causing a fuss. I couldn't discern that other people telling me I wasn't worthy and not quite good enough for them was something I shouldn't accept. To these girls, some-how I was "less than," and as a studious, obedient, Catholic grade school student, I embraced their discernment as truth.

It's funny how certain moments in our lives seep into our souls and become part of the tapestry of who we think we are and how we see ourselves for a long time afterward. I didn't have the phys-ical currency of being as cute or as charming as my friends, so my feelings of shame over my appearance caused me to accept what-ever attention they were charitable enough to offer. My feelings of unworthiness became so part of my identity that it was like I was working on earning an alternative-universe Girl Scout badge in low self-esteem.

Fast forward to 1984 when I received a phone call that changed my life and the life of my whole family. I was in the eighth grade and my sister, Kathy, who was a year older than me, had been taken to the hospital. Weeks earlier we had been out shopping at the local mall with my older sister, Ann. Ann had driven us there, so we were feeling very grown up being on our own as teens. We had stopped in the popular teen fashion store Deb, with its hot-pink sign and aisles filled with trendy fashions of thick pastel sweaters, ruffled blouses, cool neon leg warmers, and jean jackets. Stopping in front of one of the mirrored columns in the store, Kathy noticed swelling on one side of her neck. After going home and telling my parents, she went with them to a local doctor, who said it was probably an enlarged thyroid. When the issue didn't resolve itself, my parents took Kathy to the Guthrie Cancer Center in Sayre, Pennsylvania, for a second opinion. The phone call that day was my mom calling from the hospital. My sister had just come out of surgery, and my mother was calling to say she had cancer.

The news changed the trajectory of my entire family. Our routine evolved into trying to keep our usual schedule while navigating drives from our home in Upstate New York to weekly cancer treatments in Pennsylvania. When these treatments didn't work, one option was for Kathy to undergo a bone marrow transplant at the Fred Hutchinson Cancer Research Center in Seattle, Washington. Ann was a match to be the bone marrow donor, so my mom and two sisters moved to Seattle for several months while Kathy underwent treatment.

I was left at home with my dad to run the house at age 14. A responsible kid, I enjoyed taking care of people and animals. I had already volunteered at a home for the elderly since fifth grade, making weekly visits with the residents there. I also enjoying cleaning and cooking, so I didn't really think about the large increase in my responsibilities. We all had our roles to help get my sister through her illness, and we all did what needed to be done.

Looking back, I now realize that the responsibilities I covered during this time were more impressive than I ever gave myself credit for. Besides going to school, volunteering weekly at the retirement home, and continuing with my piano lessons, I cooked the meals, cleaned the house, did the laundry, went grocery shopping, and took care of the dog.

It didn't dawn on me how much of a mini-adult I had become until one day when the phone rang. On the other end were a mother and her son who seemed to be in his 20s. They had heard that my sister was undergoing a bone marrow transplant, and the mother wanted to find out more about the treatment for her other son (who was not on the call), who was sick with cancer. I walked them through the procedure and the risks, the few places that were performing the treatment in the United States at the time and answered all their questions, all the while trying to be reassuring. The son then asked my age. "Fourteen," I said. "Oh, my God!" they both exclaimed. The intensity of their response puzzled me slightly at the time. When people are faced with a life-and-death situation, they learn to just keep their heads down and do what needs to be done.

I can see now that the responsibility of caring for people, coupled with the feeling of being "less than" or unworthy, created the perfect conditions to develop an unhealthy relationship with food. I was packaged in an overweight body that had been told over and over again it needed to change, and I unconsciously took on the perspective that I must do things or look a certain way in order to earn love or friendship.

I was a freshman in college when I first became aware of this distorted perspective. A friend had stopped by my room to say hi, and I immediately launched into asking her if she needed help with anything or if she wanted me to go to the grocery store and get anything for her. She looked at me and said, "Mary, you don't always have to offer to do things for people for them to like you. They like you because they like you." The statement so shocked me that I can still feel the sensation of having the wind knocked out of me by her words, even all these years later.

The validation and acceptance that I had only consistently received from food and dogs up to that point was now manifesting itself in an authentic friendship. My friend helped me crack open a window to a world in which food didn't have to be my only true friend. I began to realize that I didn't have to reject or hurt myself to find personal connection.

The first time I seriously tried to lose weight was around my sophomore or junior year in high school (before I went to college and continued to struggle with over-restricting and then bingeing). My "why" at that time was based on external feedback. I had been told for years that the way my body looked was not acceptable, so if I changed my appearance, people would have to love me, right? In high school, I bought into the typical teen movie fantasy that as soon as I lost weight, the boys would be lining up at my door, ready to take a number like at a deli counter because I was in such demand. Much to my surprise, this was not the case.

I started out sensibly by eating salads at lunch, cutting back on portions, and walking one hour every day. After I lost about 25 pounds, my mom told me, "You can stop now." Stop? I've been told my whole life to lose weight. Why stop now? It was thrilling to finally be able to wear the clothes of my skinny sisters. One day I snuck into my sister's room and borrowed her white jean shorts, totally triumphant that I could fit into the same size as her. My senior year, people occasionally commented that I was looking a little too thin. Anger sometimes flared up internally:

How dare they say this when for years they have been telling me the opposite!

The constant dieting was very difficult to keep up. My first episode of binge eating hit when I was studying for a college-level history class. We had bought a box of a new cereal called Quaker Oat Squares that my sister and I both loved. As I ate handful after handful straight out of the box, the sweet crunch of the cereal seemed to dissolve my extreme stress on contact. I couldn't stop until I had devoured almost the whole box. My behavior shocked me, and I felt sick from stuffing myself as well as confused about why I had done such a thing.

I understand now that I was eating as a way to manage the stress and anxiety I had piled on myself in my drive to do well in school. Getting good grades was a tangible way to validate my self-worth. High marks meant I was worth something; if I didn't have that I had even less value.

The next day after my Quaker Oat Squares binge, my mom was upset that the cereal was already gone. She assumed my sister and I were both guilty, and I was too ashamed to admit I was mostly responsible.

The tug-of-war, push-pull character of eating had gone into full swing during this time. Eating equally comforted and tortured me by turns. Author Susan Burton in her 2020 memoir *Empty* perfectly describes the seductive nature of bingeing "as a way to temporarily shut everything out and exist in an altered reality defined by the loosening of restraint." (Burton 2020, 95) That's precisely how I felt during a binge. The alternate reality of existing in a place free from restriction and rules was exhilarating. Freedom felt good, and I wanted more of it.

At the time, I didn't realize that my struggles were not about the food. I blindly used food for comfort and to create small rays of happiness to break through the heavy clouds of self-imposed pressure for high performance and perfection in all aspects of my life. Bingeing held me in the moment, where I experienced freedom from all the societal rules and expectations of school, home life, and appearance. Eating or not eating became a way to manage stress and emotional pain that I couldn't articulate at the time. When you are taking care of everyone else, food is one thing that can be there just for you. What I didn't realize at the time was that I would never find satisfaction using food to fill a hungry heart.

THE CARETAKERS

I want to share my story because many of the clients I work with struggle with emotional or stress eating. One common characteristic I've noticed is, like me, these clients are often the caretakers. They are the go-to people and "rocks" whom everyone relies on in their circle of family and friends. While taking care of others is important, this starts to turn into a negative when we put other people's needs ahead of our own by default and end up sacrificing ourselves in the process. We find validation and self-worth by focusing on other people and their needs but then leave ourselves empty in the process. Food becomes an easy and acceptable treat, a way to physically fill yourself when your emotional needs aren't getting met or you're not being heard or seen. You feel burnt out by doing everything for everyone all the time, but you are so used to being in the martyr role that you have a difficult time breaking free.

DO YOU FEEL LIKE MARTHA MARTYR?

Do you find yourself putting everyone else's needs first, and you're either last on the list or not even on the list at all? Do you sacrifice yourself for the approval and acknowledgment of others? Do you feel arrogant, self-centered, or just plain uncomfortable attending to your own needs? Is it easier for you to focus on other people's lives rather than your own life? Do you sacrifice your own self-care and convince yourself you don't have time to be healthy? Has taking care of others become your unselfish "badge of honor" and the reason you can't stay committed to taking action to care for yourself? In my experience, both men and women have this tendency when they're the caretakers.

Even when we're feeling burnt out, we often feel safe in our caretaker role and find it terrifying to work on changing our own life and risk failure of not getting what we want. We get that sick feeling of self-betrayal when we know we once again gave too much of our energy and time away but feel powerless to stop the harmful cycle. We have become so used to denying our needs that we have lost sight of our authentic self.

Like me in my story, you may secretly feel unworthy of love on your own merits—that you must do things for others to earn love. I believe food is one of the few acceptable ways we treat ourselves, and it's very scary to make changes to one of the few coping tools that makes us feel safe, loved, comforted, and important.

I find that we tend to give to others what we want for ourselves. We secretly wish for someone to recognize our needs and care for us the way we care for them. We yearn for someone to believe in us and see us for who we really are. When they don't, food is there for us.

YOU ARE WORTHY: BREAKING FREE FROM YOUR EMOTIONAL "BATH FITTER"

Feeling accepted, validated, and emotionally safe along with acknowledging and believing you are really worthy to receive love and care—especially from yourself—is an important first step to changing your life. Otherwise, your excuse becomes that you can't fix yourself because other people need you too much.

Instead of ignoring your needs and stuffing yourself with food, it is important to speak your truth. This allows you to break free from what I call your emotional "bath fitter." Like a custom bath fitter, where a new acrylic tub is simply placed over your existing shower or tub with a watertight seal, you probably have spent years placing a smiling case over the top of your needs, pretending everything is OK when it's really not. Eventually, your plastic cover starts to leak as emotional eating takes over.

You can break free from your emotional bath fitter, however. When you're able to identify and acknowledge your needs, food starts to take on a different meaning. Food starts to become just food rather than the way you implement self-care.

The following chapters will guide you in regaining your balance and healing your relationship with food through self-awareness and various additional strategies. The resulting impact is that learning to listen to your inner voice naturally and gently allows you to put yourself higher on your list of priorities. You begin to realize that being on automatic pilot and ignoring your needs has been hurting your health. As you discover your inner voice, you start to make more food choices based on what you want to eat, without judgment, rather than what you think you should eat based on "food rules." You're able to start identifying your needs and accept that it's OK to work on meeting them.

This allows you to be committed to taking small steps. You accept that there will be bumps in the road, but you don't use them as an excuse to give up the minute something doesn't go as expected. You learn to embrace your imperfections and see missteps as learning opportunities to do something different the next time rather than believing yourself to be a failure and falling back into old ways. You learn how to soothe yourself with activities that don't involve food. You work on identifying the true emotional issue, which allows you to use food as nourishment and enjoyment rather than as a way to dull emotional pain.

Though you may feel anxiety and fear at times about changing your intense caretaking role, you're able to take small steps to make consistent progress over time. When you start to get off track, you avoid beating yourself up. Instead, you take steps to consciously reset healthy habits. I know it can be scary to change. Taking small steps each day will reinforce the commitment you have made to yourself and help shift your mindset to knowing yourself as worthy, loveable, and deserving.

CHAPTER 5

CHICKEN DOORS AND BRICK WALLS

No one can cheat you out of
ultimate success but yourself.
— Ralph Waldo Emerson

DO YOU KNOW WHAT A "CHICKEN DOOR" IS?

In theme parks and amusement rides, the "chicken door" is an exit near the loading platform of roller coasters and other thrill rides for those who have second thoughts. The chicken door allows for a quick escape when your brain screams, "Oh, hell no!" as you stare at the ride and decide to bolt. This got me thinking about how we all have our own chicken doors in life.

I confronted my own chicken door several years ago when deciding whether or not to enter a weightlifting competition. I started listing all the excuses in my head about why it wasn't sensible: *I would have to take time off from work. I'm not going to win anyway, so why try? I could fail miserably and embarrass myself.* Writing this book was another chicken door. The negative brain starts yapping: *I'm not a writer. What do I have to say that hasn't been said before? Would anyone be interested in how I view things?*

When I realize I'm leaning toward my chicken door to get out of things that scare or intimidate me, then I know I really should do those things, because I don't want fear making my decisions for me.

You, too, may have a chicken door when it comes to making changes in your health or nutrition. You know you should be making changes, but an excuse always comes up that gives you an out. Whether or not one admits it, fear is often the captain of a person's nutrition comfort zone.

Here are some common chicken doors when it comes to nutrition:

Fear of being judged. Since eating is one of the most personal topics, you may fear being judged or embarrassed when talking about what you eat. It's scary to admit to yourself and someone else that your habits are not supporting your goals.

Fear of change. The fear of changing current habits is common, especially when you use eating to cope with life or soothe your feelings.

Fear of failure. The fear of failure is also prevalent as you may say you want to change but secretly believe that this new effort won't work either. The fear of failure is rooted in self-doubt and that it's not OK to make a mistake and try again.

Fear of success. Surprisingly, sometimes the fear of success can also be a nutrition chicken door, especially when your life has revolved around losing weight for many years. For example, you may have had an easier time losing weight than maintaining and keeping it off. The excitement of reaching a goal is often tempered by the thought, *What do I do now?*

Change is difficult because it's uncomfortable and fear may be preventing you from taking action and achieving the healthy life you yearn for. Our inherent nature as humans is to gravitate to what is familiar and routine because then we don't have to think about or invest energy in changing our habits.

Neurologically, habits reside in the basal ganglia and brainstem. Repeated behaviors literally change the neural pathways, creating established grooves in your brain highway (Yin HH 2006). That's why we often find ourselves repeating the same pattern of behavior even though it isn't serving us well anymore. We may not like what we're doing, but when we're in the moment and feeling overwhelmed, it's really hard to change our course of action. Think of it like driving to work. If you've worked at the same place for years, you probably don't have to think about the route anymore. Maybe at first you had to use your GPS to make sure you didn't miss a turn. After a few months, however, the drive likely became so automatic that you could mentally check out and arrive at work wondering how you even got there.

I have struggled with change as well and my fear prevented me from taking action for many years. For example, years ago when I was working for the federal government as a budget analyst, a coworker there threatened to quit every week. He would periodically submit his resignation letter to human resources and then pull it back at the last minute before it took effect. He did this for several years and never followed through. As I watched his chicken dance, I knew I was secretly doing my own chicken dance as well by not moving forward. I was not happy with what I was doing at the time, but I lowered my head and kept working. I convinced myself that while I might not be excited about the work, it was a stable job, and I was making a good income, so I should stay put.

During that time, I periodically binged on pizza, Pop-Tarts, and sleeves of mini doughnuts at night that left me puffy and sick with a food hangover the next day. I was so determined to make this sensible job work that I didn't make the connection between my misery at the job and binge eating as an escape from forcing myself to do something I really didn't want to do. During this time, I had been thinking of changing careers but it took me about 10 years of thinking about doing something in nutrition before I pulled the trigger and acted on changing my life. The fear of changing careers and the work to get there overwhelmed me, but eventually I was so miserable that I hit what I call my brick wall. I backed myself into a corner, and change felt like my only option if I wanted to be happy again.

> *Brick walls are there for a reason. The brick walls*
> *aren't there to keep us out. The brick walls are there*
> *to show us how badly we want something.*
> — Randy Pausch

The other day while I was waiting for an appointment, I was thumbing through a popular women's health and fitness magazine. An article that caught my attention was written by a woman who had just gone through a bad breakup with her boyfriend. As she wallowed in Häagen-Dazs ice cream and self-pity, her dad put it all in perspective: "I guess relationships have an expiration date." It was then that the woman realized she had held onto her boyfriend longer than she should have and that, like sour milk, it was time to throw out the toxic substances in her life and re-emerge healthier and happier (cue the inspirational music).

This got me thinking about the nutrition habits in our life. We may be clinging to unhealthy habits because they're as comfortable as an old pair of sweatpants. Though we may perceive that it's easier to keep doing the "same old, same old" with our eating, eventually we start to notice that we're paying a price for our habits—whether that be not looking how we want, not feeling as well, or having health problems. (Think back to having to put on a pair of pants with an actual zipper after being in quarantine for several months during the pandemic. I feel constrained just thinking about it.)

You may finally reach a point like I did at my job where you hit the brick wall—where you feel so unhappy, frustrated, discouraged, or miserable in your current situation that you can't stand it anymore. You may feel like a square peg shoved into a round hole. You intuitively know you're not honoring your true self and you've reached a dead end. *No more*, you say. *That's it. I've had it. I'm done.* You realize your only option is to change in order to free yourself.

While we may think of hitting a brick wall as a negative thing, the image I see in my mind is a bright yellow explosion with the word "Pow" written in cartoon letters, like when the superhero is defending themselves against the villain. Working on destroying this brick wall allows us to create a new path to follow our vision and rewrite our stories. In doing so, we are literally letting our light out. This creates an opportunity for freedom, growth, and renewal as we listen to ourselves and follow what we really want.

In her 2006 book, *Eat, Love, Pray*, author Elizabeth Gilbert eloquently describes this universal experience that impacts many of us, even those without food issues.

> We all want things to stay the same. Settle for living in misery because we're afraid of change, of things crumbling to ruins. Then I looked around to this place, at the chaos it has endured—the way it has been adapted, burned, pillaged and found a way to build itself back up again. And I was reassured, maybe my life hasn't been so chaotic, it's just the world that is, and the real trap is getting attached to any of it. Ruin is a gift. Ruin is the road to transformation.

Think about what your chicken door might be.

Do you worry about being judged for your food choices? Have you been in a situation where you felt self-conscious eating what you really wanted, so you made a different choice (like my story where I refused to order dessert when eating out because I was overweight and felt I didn't deserve it)? Is this fear causing you to eat in secret or not honor what you really want to do?

Do you fear changing an eating habit because it provides comfort and security?

Years ago, a friend underwent gastric bypass surgery. She lost weight and met her goal but was having a difficult time emotionally because she physically couldn't soothe herself with food the way she used to. She was forced to confront all the uncomfortable emotions she had been using food to hide from, which led her to develop healthier coping skills.

If weight loss hasn't worked for you before, do you think you're secretly doomed to fail before you even get started? You might be worried about feeling uncomfortable as you change your habits or be feeling grief or loss of a lifestyle that you know needs to change if you want your life to change. I felt this way after I lost weight in high school only to gain twice as much in college. The thought of returning to my strict eating regimen of salads and SlimFast left me feeling defeated and empty and that I needed to suffer to achieve what I wanted.

Fear of success might also be a concern. If you've spent your whole life focusing on weight loss, you might unconsciously feel that the persona of the constant dieter has become part of who you are. What would life be like without that? How would you use the resulting freedom to focus on something else?

Often, we envision becoming instantly transformed when we reach a certain size, shape, or weight. We think everything will suddenly be better, like how I thought the boys would be lining up in high school when I lost weight. But that image of what I thought my life would become did not materialize. The feelings of unworthiness and low self-esteem were still there, just in a differently shaped body.

After reflecting on your chicken doors, ask yourself the following question: Which of my lifestyle habits are way past their expiration date? Like sour milk, what patterns need to be discarded so I can remove my limits and start my transformation?

Awareness is the first step before true change can begin. The following chapters will show you steps to keep moving forward.

CHAPTER 6

KNOWING YOUR WHY

Once I made a decision, I never thought about it again.
— Michael Jordan

Before embarking on any major change in life, knowing why that change is important to us is key to our success. Too often we start doing things because we think we should—"I should lose weight," "I should eat healthier," "I should exercise"—and the list goes on. However, "should" statements are associated with guilt and obligation rather than voicing what we really want. Superficial "should" reasons never lead to lasting change because they aren't reflective of our authentic selves. We have to find the deep-down, soul-shaking reason that is so important to us that there is no other option but to change. Our "why" must honor our inner voice and vision.

Our core reason for change needs to originate from a place deeper than external influences such as work, family, friends, and negative self-talk. Listening to our inner voice helps to separate the "should" from what we really want. Clearing away the noise helps bring a clarity to our purpose and, ultimately, a commitment to action that is undeterred. We need to be so dedicated to our "why" that we decide we are going to act no matter what other distractions arise, that we will not be derailed.

The road will not be perfectly smooth with sunshine and roses. Nope, like everything in life, we will be faced with bumps along the way. But when the bumps rise up—and yes, they will find our path—we don't use them as an excuse to quit. We look for a way to work around them instead of giving up. We extend ourselves the grace to be imperfect, to allow ourselves to keep focusing on the destination rather than the bumps.

> *He who has a why to live can bear almost any how.*
> — Friedrich Nietzsche

Let's revisit for a minute my program analyst work for the federal government. The job "should" have been a good fit for me because I had gone to school for political science and had an interest in government, but as time went on, I started to ask myself, *Do I really want to do this for the rest of my life?*

From fifth grade through high school, I had volunteered at a home for the elderly, visiting the residents there. Later, in my adult job, I missed seeing the direct impact of helping others that I had experienced in my youthful volunteer work. Plus, I wasn't excited or passionate about my program analyst responsibilities. In an attempt to quell my unhappiness, I binged on sweets and fast food until I finally reached a brick wall of self-imposed suffering. At that point, I sat myself down and asked, *If I had a magic wand and could anything I wanted, what would I do?* My immediate answer was that I would talk to people about their nutrition. My struggle to become healthy and fit as an adult was sparking a passion to return to school to help others. I decided that becoming a dietitian was the best educational path for me.

To achieve my goal, I returned to school to earn a bachelor's degree in nutrition. With no science classes under my belt, I had to start from scratch. First, I took as many classes as I could at the community college. I applied to a few four-year schools, but the one that was closest would have cost out-of-state tuition, which I couldn't afford. I chose a great in-state school, but it was a solid two-and-a-half-hours' drive away from my home. Classes weren't offered online, and it had a traditional program structure, so I quit my job and for two years drove back and forth to school several days a week in order to get that degree. Moving closer to school wasn't an option at the time.

After taking one of my first classes at the new school, I stood in the parking lot and started to cry, overwhelmed by thoughts of being separated from family, driving hours a day, and being the oldest student in my classes. My rational brain questioned my decision: *What am I thinking? Are all these sacrifices really worth this stress?* But my heart kept my questioning brain in check. My passion for my "why" along with the strong desire to change my life and do what I truly wanted to do prevented me from allowing fear to make my decisions. I was so devoted to my "why" that I was determined to figure out a way to make my vision happen, no matter how much discomfort the process brought me. My hope and passion for helping others and changing my life in the process kept me going during these times of fear and doubt.

I've seen the same kind of determination in my most success-ful clients—people who are going through divorces, working sev-eral jobs, dealing with illness. The common thread for each one is that when they walked into my office, they had already made the decision that they were going to change their lives for the better. So when difficulty arose, they didn't throw in the towel and say it was too much—they just kept going.

One client stands out in my mind as I write. She came to see me to lose weight and improve her blood sugar numbers. Her "why" was to become healthy so she could be there for her fam-ily. Over the course of the year, she went through an unexpected divorce, earned a master's degree while raising her two young children, and dealt with one of her older sons struggling with a mental health issue. Amid all this, she lost over 40 pounds, tried new activities such as dancing and yoga, and focused on self-care. She had many valid reasons to put her health on the back burner, but she never did. I could tell she had already decided that she mattered, she was important, and she needed to put herself higher on the list if she was going to deal with all the intense issues in her life. She had a wisdom and quiet acceptance that life was difficult, but it didn't stop her from achieving what she wanted.

As you read about my story and my client's story, is your "why" for change coming into focus for you? Are you able to clear out the noise of other people's thoughts or expectations along with your own fears and doubts and listen to what you really want? Is your rational brain telling you a story that your heart agrees or disagrees with? Do you feel your choices are honoring your authentic self, or are you using food as the main coping mechanism to quiet the voices of unhappiness and discontent?

Achieving what we want often requires us to think outside the box so we can see and develop a new path that allows us to work through our challenges rather than be blocked by them. Instead of looking at a challenge and thinking, *I can't do that*, we can rephrase that internal conversation and ask, *OK, what can I do?*

As we will talk about in later chapters, the process for changing our relationship with food, and ultimately our life, requires consistent steps each day. We don't have to solve a lifetime of struggle in one day and it's not realistic or healthy to undertake extreme measures in an effort to avoid putting the work in that such a transformation requires. We need to be so committed to our "why" that we find a way to get there and keep going even when the going is more difficult than we want. The path becomes very clear when we are living our purpose and honoring our true selves. It's not necessarily easy, but speaking from my experience, it is worth it.

CHAPTER 7

THE MIRROR HAS MANY FACES

People are like stained glass windows.
They sparkle and shine when the sun is out,
but when the darkness sets in, their true beauty
is revealed only if there is light from within.
— Elisabeth Kübler-Ross

One of my childhood highlights was watching the Miss America pageant on TV. I sat transfixed on the couch in my pink bathrobe and matching pajamas ready for a late night with my two older sisters and mom. Holding a piece of paper and pencil, I prepared to write down my favorite top ten states and see how my choices compared to the judges' choices. I cringe a little now to look back and see how much I embraced the idea of rating women on a scorecard of looks and talent. But I was a good student and aiming for high scores seemed natural to my young self.

I loved watching the pageant. The sculpted, beautiful women in sparkly dresses with long, flowing hair were like bright, shiny diamonds in the sunlight, and I felt warm and happy gazing at something so seemingly perfect, beautiful, and dazzling, even if I did not feel beautiful myself. Over and over again, I had been told I was overweight or fat, which I heard as, "You are ugly, unattractive, and not good enough." The pageant contestants, on the contrary, deserved love because they had achieved a level of physical perfection so high that I only dreamed of someday climbing to the bottom rung of their platform. I did not look like the women on TV, but they gave me hope that maybe I could transform myself once I was older. If I could improve my scorecard, I knew I could be loved, too.

Like me, you might have similar stories of images on TV, in the movies, or in magazines affecting how you felt about yourself and your body, as these images did not reflect what you looked like. Some good news is that we're now seeing more inclusive images of people of all backgrounds, cultures, sizes, and shapes— as this diversity is finally being acknowledged and celebrated. However, the media and society still have a long way to go in the concept shift toward a more fully evolved understanding of what beauty is.

Society's messaging about appearance still translates into pressure-filled messages we hear all the time about food and dieting. We're bombarded with messages about self-love and internal beauty alongside headlines on women's magazines in check-out lines: "Over-40 Belly Fat Cure," "Drop 11 Pounds in 7 Days," "9 Surprising Ways to Trick Yourself into Losing Weight." In other words, love yourself, but make sure you look good, too. Feed yourself but keep yourself small. The pressure is immense. Everyone has a slightly different idea of what the "ideal" body is, and what we believe is beautiful is often a reflection of what we value.

Recently I read an Instagram post of a body-positive health coach and saw a nasty comment by a troll saying the coach was a fat piece of crap. I cringe even as I write this to relay the story. Calling someone fat is a go-to insult people use to lash out and try to devalue others. Body shaming is still a way people try to inflict hurt and damage on others. It's no wonder we feel a disconnect between what we see and how we feel about ourselves. It makes sense why these conflicting messages affect how we think about food and how we use it to try to control our bodies.

These messages foster the belief that if your body is a certain size or shape, it will protect you from being wounded.

We can really see the negative impact of these conflicting messages in how they play out in the concept of self-image. We are conditioned to be critical of our appearance and are constantly trying to figure out ways to "fix it" with diet and exercise. But it's not really about the food; it's about the belief that we must control our bodies to achieve an acceptable appearance. We often look in the mirror and see only what we perceive as flaws. No wonder what we think we see in the mirror is usually not an accurate reflection of reality, regardless of our size.

An example of this disconnect is often witnessed in a therapeutic exercise called body tracing. Body tracing is a technique that compares a person's perspective of their body with a verified version. It involves first drawing what you think the outline of your body looks like and then comparing it to an actual tracing of your body on pieces of butcher block paper. The purpose of this exercise is to foster greater self-awareness and discussion as you explore the concept of body image.

The experiment usually results in radically different images as people draw themselves in distorted sizes and shapes compared to their actual body. Many people fear that the tracing is going to be much larger than the image they draw freehand, and they are often shocked at how much smaller they are in reality than they perceive themselves to be. Body tracing can feel like an optical illusion; you continue to believe in your misperception of a skewed image even though rationally you're faced with the truth that it's not accurate.

What makes a person's vision so distorted? What makes a person believe and cling to ideas about his or her body that aren't true?

How we see ourselves is much more than the physical image we see in the mirror. Our self-perception is based on our mind's eye, how we feel about ourselves and our interpretation of others' perception or feedback given to us. It's influenced by our life story— what has happened in the past, what our current circumstances are, and how we view our future. Negative self-perceptions cause stress, depression, and anxiety. Guilt that comes from disappoint-ment that we haven't "fixed" ourselves yet usually fosters feelings of shame as we tell ourselves we are weak and flawed. Food then becomes a tool we use to "punish" ourselves because of internal-ized messages that we are not worthy.

Who is the person you see in your mind's eye versus the one you see in the mirror? Do you feel it matches up, or is there a dis-connect? Is this vision of yourself something you have believed for a long time? When did you start seeing yourself this way? Was there a specific memory or moment that created this per-ception? Do you think this is still true? Do you focus only on physical aspects you feel you need to change? If so, do you use food to punish yourself based on what you see in the mirror?

In the next chapter, we will continue exploring the impact of our perceptions of ourselves and our internal dialogue upon our food choices and turn toward the importance of creating a positive future vision to focus on. Instead of using food to punish ourselves, we can use food to fuel our bodies in an empowering way that gives us the energy we need to accomplish our vision. We want to learn to choose food that is pleasing to us and that honors how it makes us feel.

The later chapter on mindful eating helps us learn how to bridge the gap between doing what we feel we "should" do and listening to ourselves. Mindful eating helps to put food in a better balance and perspective so that food becomes food again. Then we don't use food to hurt ourselves because others have hurt us or because we feel "less than" or unworthy; we use food to fuel ourselves in a loving and nurturing way. Mindful eating allows us to end the battle with food so we can heal ourselves.

CHAPTER 8

THE CRYSTAL BALL: ENVISIONING YOUR FUTURE SELF

Be there for others, but never leave yourself behind.
— Dodinsky, author, *In the Garden of Thoughts*

THE CINDERELLA COMPLEX: THE SHOES HAVE IT

I've always been drawn to the concept of transformation. I used to love watching the reality TV makeover shows in which people's hair, wardrobe, or home was magically transformed in a span of 60 minutes or less. There's something so appealing about a fairy tale-like commando team of professionals swooping in and fixing all the things you've been struggling with. Don't like your hair, makeup, house, wardrobe, or life? Relax. We've got you covered.

The idea that we have the power to transform our lives if we're not happy with who we are or what our life is like holds both power and mystery. Makeover shows remind us that such change is possible. *If these people are doing it*, we think, *so can I.* For me, every phase of my life feels like it requires a slightly different version of myself as I work on executing a new vision.

Growing up, I created a version of myself that was unique from that of my two sisters. My oldest sister, Ann, was a talented artist and displayed an incredible connection with special-needs children. My sister Kathy, a year older than me, was a beautiful and multifaceted dancer in ballet, jazz, and modern dance as well as a brilliant writer. I differentiated myself by playing the piano, singing in the school choirs, volunteering at a home for the elderly, and, funnily enough, cleaning our house. In seventh grade, I received a pink feather duster as a Christmas present. I even have a picture of me holding it up joyfully after tearing open the package.

Later on, I considered going into music therapy, but in high school my interest in government blossomed and I decided to attend college in Washington, DC, to study political science. I interned on Capitol Hill and started working for the federal government when I graduated. I never played sports or was athletic in any way and didn't get into any kind of fitness beyond walking until I was in my 20s. My journey to lose weight and find a better relationship with food was what fostered the creation of a new version of myself interested in fitness.

One thing that seemed to signal each new direction in my life and offer a preview of the next version of myself was a specific change starting from the ground up—the purchase of a new pair of shoes.

Shoes often define who we think we or aren't. From kindergarten until eighth grade, I wore uniforms at the Catholic school I attended. There, one of the few symbols of individuality was a person's shoes. In the small town where I lived, a huge shoe store and the only one in town, Nolan's Shoes and Sporting Goods, spanned a large block on the main downtown street. We always parked in the back lot and climbed a steep staircase, ascending into the sporting goods section. A large kayak hanging from the ceiling perplexed and enthralled me by the way it seemed to defy logic as it dangled in the air beside the steep and scary open staircase. At the top of the steps, we'd take a right and head for the shoe section. What made the store unique was its divisions according to age group. The first section, up a slight ramp, was for babies and toddlers. The next was for school-age children. And the next for adults. You could literally feel yourself growing up as you walked a little farther up the ramp every few years and graduated from one room to the next.

Each year, it was a treat to discard the old, scuffed shoes from the past and pick out a new pair to start the school year with. I loved the whole process: First, the shoe salesman would bring out the metal foot-measuring Brannock Device that looked like a strange elongated foot. I'd stand up and carefully place the heel of my socked foot against the metal heel cup, the marked lines showing how much my foot had grown from the year before. The salesman would then slide the metal pointer on the left to my arch and the movable width bar on the right to calculate the perfect shoe size. There was something so appealing about being measured in such an exact fashion—a complex math calculation that could determine exactly who you were and what you needed. For me that meant a pair of light gray suede saddle shoes with a dark blue overlay. The style was very popular at the time and the excitement of starting a new school year was as intoxicating as the smell of a new pair of shoes, pristine in their box, laid out in the dining room along with my other school supplies of freshly sharpened pencils and crisp, new notebooks ready for the first day.

Each new pair of shoes signified a fresh start, and the style I chose each time was a reflection of who I was as well as whom I wanted to be.

Fast-forward to many years later, and shoes still played a special and meaningful role during a transformational part of my life. Over twelve years ago, when I had just finished my school and training to become a dietitian, I decided to start my own business and work for myself. Part of the process of setting up the business was to reevaluate who I was and the image I wanted to project as I started my second career. Included in my reinvention process was revising and revamping my clothes so they reflected who I was striving to be. A symbolic shoe purchase during this time was part of the future vision of myself. I was shopping with a friend who, at the time, also worked as a stylist. It was helpful to have someone envision a new me and bring that vision out by helping me make different clothing choices. We were shopping at a high-end department store looking for a pair of shoes to complete some dresses I had purchased. I don't think I would have been brave enough on my own to try some of the fancier shoes, but her encouragement made me feel more confident.

It was then that it happened. I fell in love with a pair of shoes named Sharon.

Sharon was a style of Giuseppe Zanotti patent leather peep-toe pumps. Sharon came in a variety of colors but the one I chose (or maybe chose me) was the glossy, deep brown patent leather goddess that shone with the suggestion of a subtle leopard print marked by faint golden swirls. The pin-thin stiletto heels were balanced by the platform sole under the toe that made walking surprisingly more comfortable than the style suggested. Although they were on sale, they were the most expensive shoes I had ever bought. For a woman into working out who usually made very sensible purchases, were these the most practical shoes? Of course not! But you don't choose Sharon to be practical; you choose Sharon because that's the vision of whom you want to be—strong, fun, sexy, a little daring, and beautiful, a bolder new version of myself to match my new career endeavor.

While I have to admit I haven't worn Sharon recently, I still keep those shoes in their original box and lovingly looked at them while writing this. Sharon reminds me that I changed my life. I hope Sharon's story reminds you of the importance of believing in a sense of possibility—that there is something to look forward to in the future and that you can change your life if you're not where you want to be right now.

Years ago, I used shopping to manifest the vision of my future self or future life manifested. Physical objects, such as shoes, clothes, or accessories, are ways to motivate, visualize, and implement the best versions of our current or future selves. These all set the tone for how we feel about ourselves and how we want others to perceive us. So many times, I have stood in a dressing room, trying on outfits, and fallen in love with particular items because of how they made me feel.

For me, a new outfit bolsters my confidence to show up in the world the way I ideally want to. Sometimes I've bought a dress with no particular event or place to go to, because I felt that somehow by buying it, the dress would give me the motivation to create the life that would give me a place to wear it. Sometimes buying a new workout outfit is just what we need to feel confident enough to try a new exercise class. Every time I purchase new running shoes, my desire to run soars because of the possibility of improvement. The shoes make me different.

Changing our appearance also helps to set our intention and define our next version of ourselves. Making a dramatic change to our hair by cutting it short or changing its color is often how we make a statement to the world that we are different internally. I'll never forget that iconic scene in the movie *Waiting to Exhale* in which Angela Bassett's character, Bernadine, insists that her friend chop off her long hair into a short pixie cut to signify a new determined fierceness to start putting her needs first after her husband leaves her.

Of course, it's always a balance between expressing our individuality and strengthening our self-image through outward appearance versus fostering an unhealthy obsession with body image. That's why it's so important to love the *process* of getting to a goal as much or even more than the result itself. For example, many of my clients have a weight goal in mind when focusing on weight loss. This can serve as motivation but can also cause an unhealthy mindset if a person is only focused on the number. We need to measure progress in many ways. How do we feel? Is our energy improved? Are we sleeping better? Are we getting physically stronger from new movement patterns? Are we feeling happier about our relationship with food?

You can also use visualization to create images of what you want to see in your life. Using vision board exercises to do this has become very popular. Vision boards free up our rational left brain by creating a collage of pictures and words on paper to help us envision the future we want to create. Making art allows our subconscious thoughts to be revealed by using the creative right portion of our brain. Instead of rationalizing away why something is not possible, we let go and allow new insights to float to the surface. I encourage you to explore vision boards as a way to visualize your best self.

THE MIND'S EYE: PERFECT VISION

In addition to physical objects such as our shoes or clothes to help our vision of our best selves come to life, mental imagery is also a powerful tool for changing our habits and ourselves. Mental practice has actually been found to be as effective as physical practice (LeVan 2009). Athletes use mental imagery to visualize kicking a field goal or crossing the finish line first. Gymnasts do mental run-throughs of their routines as a virtual practice or mental rehearsal to instill confidence and see themselves completing their routine successfully. Actors do a run-through of their lines while looking in the mirror as an informal dress rehearsal to prepare for the actual performance.

As we're trying to change our habits, we can use mental imagery to envision what those changes will look like and how we would implement them. For example, if we want to start exercising in the morning, we might lay out our clothes the night before, set our alarm, and imagine ourselves rolling out of bed, slipping on the outfit we set out, and opening the door to go walking. Doing this run-through in our head would help us get over the challenge of getting started, because "seeing" ourselves doing the activity—broken down into doable steps—would help it seem less overwhelming.

In terms of food, when we're hungry we use mental imagery as we think about what we want to eat and create a picture of that in our head. If we're craving pizza, we are probably visualizing what it looks like, how it smells, what it will taste like, and how it will make us feel when we finally get to eat it.

This can be a positive experience when your vision matches up with reality, but we can also be thrown for a loop when there is a disconnect between vision and reality. For example, years ago for my birthday I ate a Dairy Queen Pumpkin Pie Blizzard that was only available in the fall. Real pieces of pumpkin pie were blended in vanilla soft-serve ice cream and topped with whipped cream. The crunchy pieces of the graham cracker crust balanced the smooth ice cream perfectly. That sundae was so delicious that I thought about it for a whole year. When it finally became available again, with great anticipation I drove to the same Dairy Queen as before, ordered my sundae, and you know what? It didn't taste as good in reality as what I had imagined. While disappointed that the food I had obsessed over didn't live up to my memory of it, I quickly changed course and ordered a butterscotch-dipped cone instead.

When we truly eat mindfully, we're able to cultivate an awareness of what we want to eat, to assess if we're really enjoying what we're eating, and, if it doesn't taste satisfying, to give ourselves permission to eat something else. It's important not only to have a vision but also the ability to pivot when that vision isn't meeting our needs—whether it's a vision of what we want to eat or whom we want to become.

As we discussed in an earlier chapter, to make lasting changes, we need to not only understand our "why" but to also foster the mental flexibility to change course as we refine our vision. Having a vision of our future self provides a fantasy of a different us, a different life. It gives us a sense of possibility—something to believe in and hold onto when life is challenging. Keeping that vision in the forefront of our minds motivates us to keep going, to keep trying even when we don't want to.

While we may feel super motivated or maybe desperate to quickly change how we eat in order to transform our body and arrive at the vision in our head, there's a problem with quick fixes. They don't last. Strict diets foster the short-term brain that sees a start-and-stop pattern. We suffer through a period of restriction and then return to our usual habits. We focus on suffering for a period of time, thinking that will solve our long-term problem. We hope that the 60-minute makeover version of a diet will be the answer.

MINDFUL MARATHON: PROGRESS OVER PERFECTION

To truly change our lives, we need to transition from short-term-brain to long-term-brain thinking. Dieting is challenging but losing weight slowly and consistently by creating a balanced relationship with food serves us better in the long term by changing our foundation. Focusing on consistent small shifts that change our habits makes change more sustainable. It teaches us to eat a variety of foods that we enjoy while honoring our hunger and fullness. We learn to make better choices through mindfulness rather than restriction and deprivation. It's about making daily choices for consistent progress rather than finding the perfect diet.

For example, one client I worked with would ask herself one simple question instead of trying to change too many things at once: *Can I make a slightly better choice?* This relieved the pressure of having to be "perfect" and simplified things so she could focus on that moment in time and not worry about what happened yesterday or what might happen tomorrow. Another client wasn't ready to change any of his food choices, so we kept them the same, and he focused on tracking his eating instead and trying to be more self-aware. He lost 25 pounds in the first few months just by being more mindful about everything he was taking in.

The important thing to keep in mind with these examples is that your journey is unique to you. I always tell my clients that there are many ways to eat healthily, and it's important that we honor our specific lifestyle circumstances, what's important to us, and the pace with which we feel most comfortable moving into change. I remind my clients that while I know it's difficult to not compare our lives and progress to others', the best gift we can give ourselves is to run our own race. Since the process to achieve our vision is a marathon rather than a sprint, in the next chapter we'll talk about the importance of cultivating mental toughness to help us keep moving forward.

CHAPTER 9

JUST KEEP TRYING: THE KEY TO MENTAL TOUGHNESS

Survival can be summed up in three words—never give up. That's the heart of it really. Just keep trying.
— Bear Grylls, British survival instructor

Being outside always helps to press the reset button on my soul. I like to joke that my soul is part Goldendoodle, because I love to be outside as much as my sweet departed dog, Bella, did.

It was a beautiful fall September Sunday morning, the first weekend morning I could really feel the change of seasons—a chilly start to the day in the 40s that quickly increased to the 60s by late morning. The clear blue of the sky matched the crispness of the air, and a faint smell of burning wood wafted through the air. I was scheduled to do a long training run of 18–20 miles to prepare for my marathon next month. Everything seemed aligned—gorgeous weather, I had slept well, and my route was planned. I was wearing compression tights to help provide extra leg support and had brought my tasty refueling gels to keep my energy up during the run.

A long run has peaks and valleys not only in the route itself but in the runner's mindset. The first two miles, as I warmed up, I questioned my life choices and asked myself what in the world

I was thinking: *This seemed like a good idea when I was seated comfortably on the couch, drinking a cup of tea. Now . . . not so much.* Fortunately, I had enough experience that I could talk myself off this ledge, knowing my mood would smooth out as I ran.

I logged several miles feeling fairly strong . . . until I hit about mile 10 and fatigue started taking over my legs. The ache had begun much earlier than I had hoped, given all my preparations. My mind started racing much faster than my legs: *Ugh, I'm only halfway through this training run, and I want to stop. How am I going to make it through this run, let alone a marathon, when my legs feel like they're filled with cement right now?!*

Over the next eight miles, I cycled through several of the five stages of grief. First, denial: *Just listen to this great song. Pretend you're not even running. Hee-hee. You're just outside enjoying the day. Try not to notice that your legs are moving.* Next, anger: *I work too hard. I've done so much running this week. Why did I even sign up for this marathon?* Then bargaining: *OK, if I run two more miles, I will drink that bottle of chocolate milk sitting in my refrigerator the minute I get home.* Depression soon followed: *I feel so weak. Why is this so hard? I've been training consistently. This should be easier.* Then, finally, acceptance: *My legs are going to hurt whether I stop now or keep going. I need to get these miles in to be ready for the race. This is how the last six to eight miles of the marathon are going to feel. You need to practice feeling uncomfortable and keep going.*

> *I am thankful for my struggle because without it*
> *I wouldn't have stumbled across my strength.*
> — Alexandra Elle

Yes, the end of a marathon is the hardest. It takes every ounce of physical and mental strength to convince myself to just take one more step when all I want to do is stop. But even when I'm faced with the struggles of an intense training or race day, running frees my soul and reminds me of who I am. The ability to keep going even for just five to ten minutes more reminds me of the strength that lies inside of me.

Real strength lies in the ability to keep trying even when we have convinced ourselves we have nothing left to give. We must practice mental toughness in order to cultivate it.

TWO BRAINS ARE BETTER THAN ONE

You may have felt a similar struggle when trying to lose weight, where everything seemed to be aligned and you were ready to tackle the task at hand. You started out excited and motivated about the possibility that this time would be different. At first, you sailed along smoothly, but then changing your habits began feeling difficult much sooner than anticipated. The honeymoon phase ended, and the excitement and newness of change transitioned into the realization that weight loss is hard work that requires a consistent effort over time. Suddenly you were faced with the battle of the brains—your rational brain and your emotional brain.

The rational brain tends to be slower to respond in the moment as it analyzes the situation and tries to make a conscious decision. The emotional brain is what we consider our intuitive, or knee-jerk, reaction that responds almost instantly. In the context of food and dieting, your rational brain calmly says, *Keep focusing on making mindful choices. Eat when hungry. Get some movement to help with stress relief.* Your emotional brain, on the other hand, starts crying, *I'm so tired of focusing on weight loss. I work hard, and life is so stressful right now. I deserve a treat. I need to relax.* Our emotional brain is concerned with our feelings and our needs in the moment, while our rational brain is concerned about our long-term well-being. Together, these responses provide us with more balanced decision-making.

My rational and emotional brains love to have these types of in-depth conversations while I'm running. I actually picture these two aspects of my brain as two separate people having a conversation with each other. My emotional brain likes to sit on my right, my left brain sits on my left, and I sit in between the two. As I'm trying to analyze a situation, I will often state the opinions of each aloud like I'm the moderator in a debate. "My emotional brain feels this way," I say as I gesture with my right hand and turn my head to the right, "but my rational brain feels this way," I add matter-of-factly while I turn and gesture to my left. Acknowledging each thought as valid makes neither side of the brain right or wrong but instead helps me to better take into account various viewpoints and opinions as I analyze the situation. By listening to both, I balance the perspectives of each, since they both have valuable information to offer.

While your emotions or feelings provide a unique perspective, the rational brain can help balance out these feelings that can interfere with what you're trying to accomplish. Creating separation between the emotional and rational brains and allowing them to have conversations with each other helps to support you making balanced decisions. To differentiate between questions of the emotional brain versus the rational brain, look at the timing of the expressed worries: the emotional brain worries about today, while the rational brain worries about the impact for the future.

For example, one client told me that she really wanted a cupcake, but it was the beginning of the week and she knew she would be attending a party and eating sweets on the weekend. While her emotional brain said, *Go for it*, her rational brain said, *You've done so well making conscious choices to help support your health goals. You don't need to eat this right now. It's okay to wait until the party to eat cake.* Another client worried about trying to eat healthily while on a vacation to France. Her rational brain told her to keep following her typical diet, while her emotional brain yearned for wine, cheese, and pastries. When we discussed the situation to clarify these two perspectives, she realized that a week is not a very long time to eat differently—that it was more important to honor her emotional brain and enjoy this special moment in order to live a full life.

Holding these conversations with our "two brains" helps us honor each voice by taking into consideration their points of view and then making a mindful choice about a course of action based on experience and intuition.

WARRIOR BRAIN: MENTAL TOUGHNESS

If your brain is always carrying on these conversations, what are the intangibles or characteristics that can combine the two perspectives to help you succeed? Mental toughness seems to be the link.

Much has been written about mental toughness as it relates to sports, and a recent study (Caliper 2020) looked at what differentiates athletes drafted by the NBA each year versus hopefuls who don't make the cut. While scouts are looking for athletic potential, they're also looking for the nonphysical, or psychological, aspects of a player's game that will make them successful. The study concluded that mental toughness is not a single trait but a combination of six key factors: 1) level-headedness, 2) stress tolerance, 3) resiliency/ego-strength, 4) energy/persistence, 5) self-structure, and 6) thoroughness.

Let's look at how the traits that predict athletic success at the professional level relate to questions you can ask yourself about your behaviors, attitudes, and choices surrounding food. Like the concept of mental toughness, weight loss isn't about just one single factor; it's the compilation of behavior, attitudes, and lifestyle factors.

1. Level-headedness

Level-headedness measures how a person expresses their emotions. Individuals who scored higher remained composed in stressful situations rather than reacting more emotionally.

Level-headedness means that your emotional brain doesn't overtake all your decision-making; you let your rational brain provide input. In terms of eating, level-headedness measures your ability to regulate food temptation.

A low score of level-headedness might mean you eat to manage your emotions. You may reach for food and not even be aware of eating, because it has become such an automatic habit. If cookies or candy are in the office break room or at home, you eat them just because they are there, whether you're hungry or not.

A high score of level-headedness translates into the ability to eat when you're physically hungry rather than in response to stress, for comfort, or out of habit. You're able to eat until comfortably full, and you have food in your environment without automatically eating it. You're able to pause before reaching for food and check in with yourself to see if you're eating for physical hunger or emotional hunger.

In your relationship with food, do you have a high or low score of level-headedness? Do you tend to eat for comfort when feeling anxious, upset, lonely, or frustrated? Do you eat even when you're not hungry, just because food is in your environment?

2. Stress Tolerance

Stress tolerance relates to the effect of time and stress management on a person's ability to make self-care a priority. This trait refers to the ability to minimize worrying about possible negative consequences when faced with circumstances beyond one's control.

You might be experiencing a low stress tolerance if you feel your fast-paced and hectic schedule makes it hard for you to focus on your needs. If this is true for you, you probably tend to take care of everyone else before yourself, always moving yourself to the bottom of the list. You worry that if you don't do your usual caretaking role, people in your life will be upset with you. You may feel it's easier to shortchange yourself than risk being criticized by others.

A higher stress tolerance helps you let go of things, people, or situations that are causing you to feel drained and free up time that you need to work on your health goals. You can then focus your energy on your own self-care rather than on trying to control all situations. This might look like taking time out for exercise even when faced with a never-ending to-do list. It might mean going to the grocery store and doing some meal prepping on the weekend to have healthy foods available during the week. It might mean saying no to someone's request for help, because you would be sacrificing yourself in the process if you said yes.

Do you feel you worry about everyone else's needs more than your own? Does your busy schedule leave you so drained that you have difficulty taking care of your health? Is there one responsibility you could delegate or let go of to free up time to focus on your self-care?

3. Resiliency/Ego-Strength

The resiliency/ego-strength trait measures how well you're able to handle failure, criticism, and setbacks by how quickly you're able to bounce back and feel confident again.

A low level of this trait means you lean toward being a self-critic. You tend to measure your self-worth for the day by the number on the scale. You might solely focus on aspects of your body that you want to change. You think only about the missteps instead of celebrating small victories. If you feel you're not making progress fast enough, you might tell yourself you're a failure. You might avoid doing things because of how you look, and you might tend to isolate yourself.

A high level of resiliency, or ego-strength, means you measure your self-worth by who you are as a person instead of the size, shape, or weight of your body. You acknowledge and honor your progress, no matter how modest, because you value your ability to keep moving forward. You take setbacks in stride and don't let them totally derail you. Instead of giving up, you pause and regroup by analyzing the challenges you faced and identifying how to better navigate them in the future.

Do you judge whether you're "good" or "bad" depending on the number you see on the scale in the morning? Do you tend to focus on the parts of your body you dislike and want to change rather than reflect on the positive aspects of who you are? Are you able to define who you are without relating that definition to the shape of your body? Do you celebrate small victories or do you ignore them because you will only consider yourself successful once you have reached the end result?

4. Energy/Persistence

High levels of energy/persistence indicate you're able to sustain a high level of activity over an extended period of time when required to meet a goal.

A low level of energy or persistence might mean you have a hard time getting started. When you do start, you might give up if you don't see change happening as quickly as you want it. You might be focused on the "quick fix" solutions and lean toward extremes when dieting so you can get it over with.

A high level of this trait means you view this process as a marathon of healthy habits rather than a sprint. You make your well-being a priority and commit to taking daily action to support your overall health. You allow yourself the time to accomplish your goals rather than trying to rush through them. You embrace the journey and trust the process rather than focusing only on the end result.

Do you tend to procrastinate about making changes and constantly think, I'll start tomorrow? *Do you tend to give up easily if you think you're not making progress fast enough? Do you give yourself the gift of time to embrace the process and focus on the journey rather than only thinking about the end result?*

5. Self-Structure

Self-structure measures how well you're able to work independently and create your own work habits and methods.

In terms of food, a low level of self-structure might mean you don't have a consistent eating pattern. Some days you may forget to eat for most of the day and then eat a large meal followed by a snack at night. You might not take time to plan your meals or snacks. You might find yourself grabbing whatever you can and eating a lot of takeout or convenience foods because you feel you don't have time to deal with meal preparation.

A high level of self-structure means you decide to set aside time for meal planning. You make sure you have healthy choices available at home and work so you're not stuck eating whatever is available. You identify go-to healthy meal choices when eating out in order to give yourself options. You set up a consistent eating schedule, since fueling your body is one of the ways you honor yourself and your needs.

Do you take time to plan your meals and snacks? Do you tend to skip meals because of your hectic schedule? Do you typically order out or eat mostly packaged snacks? Is eating on a consistent basis a priority for you?

6. Thoroughness

Thoroughness refers to conscientiousness in taking full ownership of detailed tasks.

A low level of this trait tends to result in an all-or-nothing way of thinking. In such a case, you have what I call the light-switch mentality, where you're either "on" or "off" your diet—there's no in between. (We'll explore this concept of the light-switch mindset in more detail later.) You engage in restricted diets that rule certain foods off-limits and allow only very limited choices. You view your weight loss as another task with a definite start and stop on your to-do list. If you feel you aren't getting results quickly enough, you tend to blame the program or attribute it to your hectic lifestyle, which is preventing you from making progress.

A high level of the thoroughness trait means you view weight loss as making sustainable lifestyle changes. You pause and make conscious choices about food and movement by considering your options and the impact of your decisions on your goals. You ask yourself, *What can I do in this moment?* rather than being ruled by expectations in your head. For example, you fit in 10–15 minutes of walking instead of thinking it's not worth walking at all because you don't have 30 minutes. You're willing to commit to activities like journaling, meal planning, and movement rather than convincing yourself you don't have time. You take ownership of your results and embrace ways to change things to support continued progress.

Do you feel like you're either on a strict diet that eliminates certain foods or not making mindful food choices at all? Do you tend to be extremely strict as you start a diet but then find yourself giving up or burning out after a few weeks? Do you typically find that if you can't eat or exercise according to the "diet rules" in your head that you go to the opposite extreme and don't even try to make any change at all?

> The biggest wall you got to climb is the one
> you build in your mind.
> — Roy T. Bennett, author, *The Light in the Heart*

Now that we've talked about being aware of the rational and emotional brain and the traits that help you balance the two perspectives and employ mental toughness, in the following chapters we will continue to explore aspects of these concepts and how to practice habits that incorporate them into your daily life. In the next chapter, we'll talk about how your struggles with eating are not about the food—they're about training your brain and creating a new mindset that ultimately changes your relationship with yourself and how you approach eating.

CHAPTER 10

TRAIN THE BRAIN

*My whole life, people have been telling me what I could
do and couldn't do. I've always listened to 'em, believed
in what they said. I don't wanna do that anymore.*
— Rudy Ruettiger, as portrayed
by Sean Astin in the movie *Rudy*

DEFINING WHO YOU ARE:
SELF-DESTRUCTION VERSUS RECONSTRUCTION

Rudy is one of my favorite movies of all time. It's based on the
real-life story of Rudy Ruettiger, who grows up dreaming of playing football for Notre Dame even though he's too small and doesn't
have good grades or the money to attend school there. After his
best friend is killed in a steel mill accident, Rudy is determined to
leave home and make his dream happen. His journey takes him
from working his way through junior college to applying to Notre
Dame (several times) to fighting for a place on the football team
even though he's half the size of the other players. For most of his
time on the football team, he serves as a live tackling dummy and
sits on the bench until his whole team rallies around him to convince the coach to let Rudy play in the last scrimmage of the final
game because of his heart and dedication.

I love this movie because it's about perseverance. Rudy refuses to give up his dream, even when everyone tells him it's never going to happen, even when faced with challenges that most people would convince themselves they could never overcome. Rudy heard and believed the stories people were telling him until he hit the brick wall when his friend died. His friend's death was the catalyst that made him decide he wasn't going to listen to other people anymore and didn't need to believe he was powerless in his life situation. He decided he was going to listen to himself and define his life the way he wanted to.

Like Rudy, we don't need to feel powerless when it comes to our relationship with food. We may have struggled with finding our way, but that doesn't mean we're destined to struggle the rest of our lives. Making long-term, healthy changes in our relationship with food requires perseverance, especially in our mindset. As much as we need to implement daily, consistent habits, we also need to continually work on and practice strengthening our belief that we can be successful.

ARE YOU DEFINING YOURSELF FOR SUCCESS OR FAILURE?

I have worked with many people who want to make changes to their nutrition, and I can often tell who's going to be successful and who will stay stuck in their old patterns because of the stories they tell themselves about what they can and can't do or often won't do. For example, my clients will often say:

> I start off motivated to "do it right," then I start to get tired. It feels like it's way too hard.

> I've tried losing weight before, but I keep losing and gaining the same 20 pounds. It's impossible for me to lose weight.

I don't have time to walk for even 10 minutes. My lifestyle doesn't allow that. I'm too busy.

I see other people eating whatever they want all the time, and they don't gain weight. It's not fair.

I've tried to lose weight, but it didn't work. There must be something wrong with my body.

NEGATIVE SELF-TALK

These types of negative internal conversations reinforce the belief that we are powerless to change our situations. We feel guilty and stressed that we haven't been able to figure out a solution, which reinforces feeling isolated, overwhelmed, and unhappy.

We become resistant to change when we get exhausted and discouraged by the constant struggle of thinking about having to change our usual mode of behavior. In terms of eating, we then tend to ignore any positive habits and exaggerate the negative. We categorize foods according to whether we or society deem them "good" or "bad." Food becomes a moral argument rather than just food. Eating something healthy makes us worthy and virtuous, while straying off the path results in being "bad." This often leads to a cycle where one misstep can send us spiraling into an episode of binge eating, feeling that we have to eat all the "bad" foods now as we make an unrealistic silent pact with ourselves that we will never eat them again. We think strict control will solve the situation. But putting oneself in shackles has never led anyone to freedom.

WHAT IS YOUR STORY?

When I'm brainstorming with clients and they respond to each suggestion with "I can't do this" or "I can't do that," alarm bells start screaming. The sirens also start whooping when clients tell me they will only be successful if I give them a strict meal plan and direct them exactly what to eat minute by minute. We convince ourselves that we "can't" do certain things because if we tell ourselves we're not able to (for whatever reason), it gets us mentally off the hook. Or if we're not given a choice about what to eat, it takes the responsibility off us. *If I'm not successful*, we think, *it's because she told me exactly what to eat and it didn't work.* Or we might say to ourselves, *My hectic schedule makes it impossible for me to live a healthy lifestyle.* We can rationalize that it's not our fault and then justify why we are where we are.

What stories are you telling yourself that are keeping you stuck, or what are the labels or stories other people have told you that you still believe?

Running falls into this category for me. I often catch myself internally and externally saying, *I'm not a "real" runner,* because I know people who race all the time or do ultra-endurance events. I remember a conversation on social media a number of years ago where people discussed whether or not they considered themselves an athlete. What was really interesting was that many people were almost afraid to call themselves an athlete if they were going to the gym and working out consistently but not playing a specific sport at a higher level. They tended to minimize their commitment and say, "Well, I consider myself somewhat athletic but not an athlete." Using minimizing labels and language does a disservice because it doesn't honor what we are doing or who we really are. These types of labels and language give life to the voices in our mind that tell us that who we are or what we do is not enough and never will be.

So what if you call yourself a runner or athlete but someone else doesn't agree with your definition? There's always someone else who's going to be a faster runner or a better athlete than you, and there's always someone whom you're going to be faster or more athletically skilled than. So what if you've been struggling with your weight for most of your life? That doesn't mean you have to accept it as your destiny. The world has a million ways to try and crush you. Don't do it to yourself first. Instead, change your story.

The stories, language, or labels we use most constantly remind us of who we are and what our truth is. We need to use these labels intentionally to remind ourselves of who we truly are and what we are capable of accomplishing. This empowers us to change our mindset from "I can't" to "I will."

Instead of saying, "I have to," try, "I choose to."

For example, reframe "I have to go to the gym" to "I'm choosing to go move my body, so I have more energy and strength to do the things I want to do."

Instead of "I failed again," try, "What can I learn from this?"

For example, reframe "I ate cake when I wasn't really hungry, and I failed again" to "I ate cake because I was feeling stressed. The next time I feel this way, I will practice pausing by getting some fresh air to change my perspective before deciding whether or not I want to snack."

Instead of saying, "It's not fair," try, "My journey is my own."

For example, reframe "It's not fair. I saw my friend eating chips, and she doesn't seem to gain weight" to "My life is unique, and my food choices and habits are going to be different from someone else's, and that's OK."

Instead of saying, "This won't work," try, "I'll figure it out."

For example, reframe "I've tried to lose weight so many times, and this probably won't work either" to "I'm approaching losing weight differently this time. I will figure out what habits are serving me well and what habits I need to let go of to get where I want to go."

One strategy to help you change negative self-talk is to retrain your brain to look at things like you're a scientist. Observe your behavior or data with an inquisitive rather than an emotional or judgmental perspective. Scientists take many data points, analyze them, and then experiment with an action to witness the impact. For example, say you decide to weigh yourself and you see a number that triggers you into negative self-talk: *Ugh, I'm so heavy. I'm 30 pounds heavier than when I used to think I was fat. I'm such a failure.* Instead of viewing the number on the scale as a rating of success or failure, pretend you have a lab coat on and you're recording the number simply as data. Your self-talk, when viewing it without emotion, might sound something like this: *Oh, wow. That's really interesting. I think I'll experiment and add in some walking to see how that impacts this number.* You then may decide to weigh yourself a few times a week to desensitize yourself to that number as you take averages and observe fluctuations or trends over time.

The fact that this example includes weighing yourself is by no means a prescription that you need to hop on the scale, but I wanted to use this example because weighing oneself can be highly triggering for so many people. Other ways we can assess progress is by how we feel, how our clothes fit, if we increased our muscle mass, or if our lab work has improved. However you decide to measure progress, you want to create positive self-talk that helps you analyze your progress and then tinker with your habits to assess their impact.

Reconstructing habits can't happen without changing our mindset. For example, one of my clients who had struggled with emotional eating for most of her life finally experienced a breakthrough. She had been clinging to the diet mentality of restriction and labeling herself "good" when she ate what she considered healthy foods and "bad" when she ate sweets. This mindset of restriction was preventing her from eating what she really wanted at meals and, as a result, she would overeat candy and cookies to compensate for the self-imposed feeling of deprivation. We worked together, and she started eating the foods she really wanted at meals. Instead of eating a salad, she would mindfully eat the pasta she had made for her family. Listening to herself and honoring what she really wanted to eat eliminated the urge to binge on dessert, because she felt satisfied with her food choices.

I always remind clients that tuning into your internal voice steers you in a positive direction. Instead of having to compensate with more food because we feel deprived, we free ourselves up by surprisingly giving ourselves permission to eat the food we are so desperately avoiding. Honoring ourselves and our internal wisdom is the foundation that allows us to build a healthier relationship with food. Food then becomes just another positive aspect of our lives instead of our lives revolving around what we should or shouldn't eat all the time.

Retraining the brain takes work, but over time it will happen with consistency. I've seen the positive impact on my clients and my life from retraining the brain as well as from applying positive self-talk. Practicing these internal conversations helps us keep moving forward so we can reconstruct our stories and, ultimately, our lives. I'm confident you can do the same.

CHAPTER 11

TURN OFF THE LIGHT-SWITCH MINDSET: CREATING A NEW MENTAL MAP

*You need to learn how to select your thoughts just the
same way you select your clothes every day. This is a
power you can cultivate. If you want to control things in
your life so bad, work on the mind. That's the only thing
you should be trying to control.*
— Elizabeth Gilbert, author, *Eat, Pray, Love*

I often have clients who state that they tend to approach everything in their life with an all-or-nothing attitude. I call this the light-switch mindset—you're either "on" or "off"—there's no in-between dimmer settings. This mindset causes us to think in absolutes:

I can't just eat a little. I have to eat all of it.

I have no self-control. If it's in the house, I'm going to eat it.

I've blown it, so I might as well eat it all at once to get it over with.

I usually then ask them, "If you went out to the parking lot and found out you had a flat tire, would you take out a knife and slash the other three?"

I hope not.

The all-or-nothing mindset is one of the common thinking traps that often happens with ideas around food, weight, and our self-image. Officially known as cognitive distortions, these disordered thought patterns cause us to interpret reality through a clouded lens, creating irrational expectations related to eating. According to mental health expert Dr. John Grohol (2019), "Cognitive distortions are simply ways that our mind convinces us of something that isn't really true. These inaccurate thoughts are usually used to reinforce negative thinking or emotions—telling ourselves things that sound rational and accurate, but really only serve to keep us feeling bad about ourselves."

The problem with the perfectionist or all-or-nothing mindset is that it leads to nothing. Our brain makes the judgment, *Do it perfectly or it's a total failure.* None of us are perfect, yet we expect ourselves to be perfect when it comes to our nutritional choices. As soon as we make one perceived misstep, we often give up because we feel everything is ruined. The mental gavel bangs loudly, serving judgment: *You are a failure.*

I have struggled with this all-or-nothing mindset in my own life when it comes to eating. In college, I would alternate between being really strict and eating only salads, which would then send me spiraling into ordering pizza or Chinese food almost every night, followed by a trip to the vending machine for Pop-Tarts, Snickers bars, Ritz Bits crackers, and/or Honey Buns. I'd figure I had "blown it," so I might as well go and eat all the "forbidden" foods, since tomorrow I would get back on track. I would also unrealistically tell myself that I would never eat these foods ever again. I got stuck in a loop that had no middle ground.

This perfectionist mindset also sets up a pattern of self-sabotage. You wait for all the conditions to be perfectly aligned before you attempt to start anything. For example, when a client and I were talking about adding in some walking for movement, the client said, "I'll start on Monday." Since we were meeting on a Tuesday, this meant she was planning to wait almost a week before taking action. For many people, Monday is the "clean slate" day where they can start fresh. This mindset has often been instilled in us from a young age. It's that feeling of starting fresh and new, like new pages in a notebook, except you write one word, decide it's not perfect, and then rip the page out and go to the next. Suddenly you have a notebook with only a few pages in it but not much to show for the missing pages.

Many people with food issues are weighed down by stories from their growing-up years that have fostered this all-or-nothing mindset and that still affect them today. For example, many clients I work with struggle with bingeing on sweets. One client shared that when she was growing up, her mother would hide any kind of sweets and desserts from her, terrified that her daughter would become fat. This resulted in the client bingeing on cookies and candy, unable to limit herself to small portions. These episodes would then lead to weeks, and sometimes months, of binge eating. By working together, we were able to change this pattern of behavior by addressing the root cause. It wasn't about the sweets. It was about the mindset of restriction and deprivation. The fact that this food had been declared forbidden drove my client to hoard or binge on as much as she could while she had a chance, even as an adult. The fear of loss, not necessarily the food itself, was driving her choices.

Sometimes when you are struggling with "forbidden food," the best thing is to give yourself permission to eat a forbidden food every day. That doesn't mean unlimited portions, but if you give yourself permission to eat it today, tomorrow, and the next day, suddenly it's not such a big deal. You start to learn that you don't have to make "perfect" choices to make progress. *The way to become more flexible is to make room for deviation.*

DIMMER SWITCH

Years ago, I worked with another client who would try to eat "perfectly healthy" at the start of the week but would then get to Wednesday and binge on ice cream. So as part of the plan, we had her eat a portion of ice cream every single day. First, this retrained her brain; since she had permission to eat ice cream, it wasn't such a big deal anymore. As time passed, the need to eat unlimited portions tended to dissipate.

Secondly, the ice-cream-every-day schedule demonstrated that she didn't need to have an all-or-nothing approach when it came to nutrition. One perceived "bad" food doesn't make a person unhealthy, and eating one perceived "good" food doesn't automatically make someone healthy either. Part of balanced eating is knowing how to include treats as part of one's overall intake.

I compare this mindset to budgeting. If we're trying to save money, does that mean we're never to go shopping again? No, we just want to cover our base bills first and then see what we have left to play with. It's the same thing with eating. We still want to have what I call our foundational foods to meet our nutritional needs, but that doesn't mean we can't have some "fun foods" as well. Fun foods are foods that typically don't have a lot of nutritional benefit to offer for the investment but are foods we eat just because they taste good to us. Fun foods tend to be sweets such as candy, cookies, cakes, pies, and ice cream; snack foods such as chips and crackers; and fast food. Fun foods can definitely be part of healthy eating, but they can cause issues when we focus on them exclusively or use them, as I did, to quiet difficult emotions.

A NEW MENTAL MAP

Giving yourself permission to eat certain foods helps to create a new mental map of how to navigate your choices and feel
good in the process. It frees you up to aim for progress, not
perfection. The journey is then filled with flexibility, balance, and
a self-compassion that is supportive of your physical and emotional health.

CHAPTER 12

ACKNOWLEDGE EMOTIONS

In Louisiana, one of the first stages of grief is eating
your weight in Popeyes fried chicken.
— Ken Wheaton, author, *Sweet as Cane, Salty as Tears*

Food is one of the most pleasurable experiences we have in life, but it can also become a source of pain when we use it exclusively to manage our feelings. Vivid memories remind me of the pleasurable and painful duality of food.

I used to take art lessons with my older sister on Saturday morning. One wintry morning, my dad picked us up after class and took us to a small cafe for hot chocolate and doughnuts. It was a treat to go out for something as regular as hot chocolate when my dad was the one picking us up instead of my mom. The cafe's bistro-style wooden table felt like a balancing act as I perched on a chair tall enough that my short, little legs couldn't reach the foot rungs. I felt like one of those bears dancing on a ball in the circus while carefully sipping the hot liquid, trying not to spill it. The hot chocolate came in a clear glass, so I could study the line between the cocoa and the large dollop of real whipped cream that magically floated on top, decorated with delicate curls of chocolate. The sweetness of the cocoa intensified the sugary taste of the doughnut, and the warmth of the hot chocolate coupled with the coziness of cuddling in my puffy winter jacket with my family around me felt like a protective barrier against the cold world. It was a sweet moment in so many ways.

Contrast that experience to years later when I was living with a close friend in my first apartment after graduating from college. I was a late bloomer, and it was the first time I'd had a boyfriend. The stress of trying to navigate being on my own while dealing with a challenging first relationship made me revert back to seeking comfort in all my forbidden fun foods such as baked goods, ice cream, and pizza. Adding to the stress was the fact that my roommate's boyfriend had done a de facto move-in; while he didn't officially live with us, he was there every waking moment. I used to hide in my room as a way to avoid confronting the situation. (I didn't reach my breaking point until her boyfriend suggested that "we" should subscribe to ESPN . . . and I didn't watch sports.)

My then-boyfriend had visited earlier in the afternoon, toting over two dozen Krispy Kreme original glazed doughnuts along with him since the boxes were buy one, get one free. I grew up in Upstate New York and was unfamiliar with the cult following of the Krispy Kreme brand until I moved to Virginia. It was then that I learned about the iconic "Hot Now" neon-red light that glowed when fresh, hot doughnuts were being churned out on the conveyor belt. My boyfriend was extremely active and skinny and he immediately scarfed down several doughnuts as a meal. I had lost weight after college and I remember just staring at him in a mix of envy and disbelief that he could eat so many doughnuts in one sitting. He quickly lost interest in the doughnuts, however, and ended up leaving the rest of them in my apartment. Later that night, while hiding alone in my room feeling isolated and unhappy, I started eating the sweet, glazed confections. Doughnuts were a forbidden food, and my reserve held out for only so long. Once I started eating, the soft, gooey stickiness of the glazed dough melted in my mouth, and I couldn't stop eating until I had easily finished off a dozen. What had started as a sweet distraction had turned into feeling stuffed and sick as I graduated from the doughnuts to cake and cookies; since I was feeling miserable already, I figured I might as well go for it and get in all my forbidden foods before I put myself back in lockdown. As I ate, I told myself I would never eat such things again.

For me, bingeing was a way to treat myself and meet emotional needs that weren't being met. Bingeing can be very appealing because it puts a person into a trance-like state where they stuff and stuff themselves even though they're physically uncomfortable. Similar to drinking, it's about letting go and losing oneself in the moment while having the thrill of being out of control. Having a perfectionist mindset gives us a high when we're "in control" and eating what we consider a "perfect" diet, but the pressure to continue this restriction is immense. Though bingeing makes a person feel physically sick afterward, the mental release from the self-imposed diet rules is liberating when they're in the moment of "freedom."

Even if binge eating is not an issue for you, you might have grown up where food was used as a reward: Eat your dinner and you can have dessert. Win your softball game and go out for ice cream. Get good grades and have a special dinner out.

Food might have also been used as a way to show care and affection or to comfort you: Scrape your knee and get a cookie. Experience a breakup and indulge in chocolate.

Years ago, one of my clients recounted a story of her cat throwing up on her bedspread, after which her first thought was, *I need chocolate.* We both had a good laugh, because we've all been there: Something stressful happens, and you seek comfort in food even though it does nothing to address the real issue.

There's nothing wrong with using food for reward or comfort. This is a natural and healthy part of our human experience. The problem is when food becomes our everything—the main way we manage our emotions and one of our only sources of pleasure. It becomes a temporary fix that can have lasting negative consequences.

Figuring out when you transition from a healthy to unhealthy reliance on food for comfort can be challenging at times, but here are a few things to consider. Reaching for a few cookies after a meal and eating a portion that makes you feel satisfied and positive is part of balanced eating. Reaching for cookies automatically anytime you feel stressed, upset, anxious, or bored can signal that you're relying too much on food as a coping mechanism. Being mentally "checked out" and not even really tasting or enjoying what you're eating can be another sign of overreliance on food, along with feeling compelled to eat a large portion even though you aren't physically hungry and mentally don't even want the food anymore. Often this leads to negative impacts of physically feeling too full, fatigued, and sluggish along with more stress, guilt, and regret as eating doesn't address the real issue and you feel defeated by your actions. Overreliance on food for comfort can result in a body weight we're not happy with, along with health issues such as high cholesterol, blood sugar, and/or blood pressure.

In a 2010 *Washington Post* health article, columnist Jennifer LaRue Huget (2010) wrote about what she learned on her journey to lose 10 pounds by her fiftieth birthday. It was so much more than about how to lose weight. Huget realized that when you can no longer use food as a security blanket to shield you from the challenges of life, you're forced to confront what you were using food to try and hide from. "That means having the unsettling discussions you'd been avoiding, fighting the fights you'd just as soon have skipped. It means sitting down at the computer and doing your work instead of buying time with a big bowl of popcorn. It also means staring down fears, working to resolve nagging problems instead of hushing them with a chocolate bar."

I love this last sentence because I think it's so true. How many times have you found yourself eating something—that you weren't even really tasting—out of habit or as a way to cope? We've all had the experience of waiting for our meal at a restaurant and mindlessly eating bread or chips and salsa just because it was sitting on the table in front of us. This brings to mind one Christmas where I hid in the living room, sat on the couch, and ate almost an entire tin of Royal Dansk Danish Butter Cookies just because they were available. I downed cookie after cookie even though they didn't even taste good after the first few. I "never" ate cookies, so this was my chance to indulge. The only reason I didn't polish off every single cookie was the anticipatory shame that my family would be asking where all the cookies had disappeared to. If I left a few among all the white papers in the tin, it might give the impression that other people had eaten them as well.

It's easy to turn to food for temporary satisfaction or distraction because it's so widely available and acceptable. Food is everywhere—in the break room at work, at convenience stores when you stop to get gas, at gyms that offer pizza nights to encourage you to join. One client told me about a coworker who would fill a glass candy jar on her desk with M&M's every day. As the distinctive clinks echoed throughout the office, coworkers' heads would pop above the walls of their cubicles like meerkats popping up out of a hole. Food-delivery services are a big business as well. In my day, Pizza Hut delivery was the only option. Now a person can get everything delivered from fast food to doughnuts to groceries.

The challenge this convenience brings is that we become conditioned to using food as our coping mechanism rather than addressing the real issues in our lives. We become so accustomed to automatically reaching for a cookie or chips when we're happy, sad, bored, stressed, lonely, upset, or distracted that it's hard to know when we're really physically hungry versus emotionally hungry. A client told me about one time she didn't even realize she had eaten candy and was perplexed when she looked down at her desk and saw it littered with candy wrappers.

IF FOOD CALLS YOUR NAME, YOU DON'T HAVE TO ANSWER

If you struggle with using food to manage your feelings and cope with your emotions, I recommend the book *The Emotional Eater's Book of Inspiration* by Debbie Danowski. This book provides 90 funny and poignant truths about overcoming food addiction.

According to Danowski, when we don't want to experience our feelings, we turn to food to help us feel better. Somehow the notion of hunger gets lost in a sea of emotions, and we forget why we're eating in the first place. We then become disconnected with our bodies and what true hunger feels like. Using food to cope creates a new host of problems and doesn't address the original issue. When the ice cream in the freezer is calling out to you, "Come and get me," Danowski suggests remembering, "Despite what we may think, food cannot speak to us. It does not breathe. It is not living, and we cannot hurt its feelings if we don't eat it" (Danowski 2007, 15).

Danowski goes on to discuss how we become emotionally attached to food by creating a human relationship with it. When I happened to see a t-shirt someone was wearing in the gym—"Chocolate doesn't ask silly questions. Chocolate understands."—I was reminded of her concept that we give human characteristics to food. I laughed when I saw the shirt, because we all have those certain foods that we feel are our friends. We know that life and people can disappoint us, but food is always there. The question to reflect on is, *Am I using chocolate occasionally for comfort, or has my relationship with chocolate become more important than the one I have with myself or other people?*

Our interactions with people in social settings make our relationship with food even more complicated. In my experience, for people pleasers and caretakers, socializing creates an environment that makes it difficult to resist overindulging because of the tendency to seek the approval and acceptance of others. A 2012 (Warner) study conducted at Case Western Reserve University validated this. The study showed that people pleasers tended to overeat at parties in an effort to make other people feel more comfortable by matching what those other people were eating. People pleasers were more likely to give in to pressure to eat more, because they perceived that the other people would feel threatened if they did not eat.

So if you're reading this and realizing that chocolate or some other food has become your best friend, or that you're eating something just to satisfy someone else, how do you reconnect to physical hunger when your emotions have been in charge of your food choices and eating habits for so many years?

FOOD FOR THOUGHT: CULTIVATING CONSCIOUS EATING

Mindful Eating Journal

The first step to changing our habits is becoming aware of them. I encourage you to keep a journal—whether you just put pen to paper or track with an app or in an online document—to become aware of what you're eating, when you're eating, how fast you're eating, why you're eating, and how you feel about your choices. Here are the key elements to capture.

How Empty Is Your Cup? Assessing Your Physical Hunger before Eating

On a scale of 1–10—with 1 being you're ready to gnaw on the table and 10 being Thanksgiving full—how hungry are you? Ideally you want to be around 4–5 in terms of hunger. You may notice your stomach growling or an empty feeling. It's been a few hours since you had a meal or snack. You're ready to eat but not so hungry that you feel light-headed or are so overwhelmed with hunger that you can't think. You may have become so accustomed to eating at certain times or on a certain schedule that you have forgotten to pause and pay attention to your body's physical cues.

Other clients state that they never feel hungry. They can go for most of the day without eating. Are you someone who doesn't feel hunger? You may have lived for years as a high performer, being so busy at work or at home that you don't even think about eating or drinking. You don't take time out to fuel your body and, as a result, you don't even feel hunger anymore. Rating your hunger can help you get back in touch with your body to enable you to pay attention to its signals again. Think of it like having the radio on with the same songs playing over and over again at the same volume. Like hunger pangs, you may notice the noise at first, but you get so used to hearing it that it becomes as much like background noise as the sound of the air conditioner fan kicking in. Rating your hunger is like changing the channel on the radio and pumping up the volume. It helps to heighten your awareness, so you start hearing it again.

When rating your hunger, ask yourself:

Is my stomach growling?

Does my stomach feel empty?

When was the last time I ate?

Am I feeling light-headed or low in energy?

Am I thinking more about food?

Pre-meal Emotional Temperature Check

Take note of the emotions you are feeling before you start eating. Are you stressed, bored, lonely, tired, frustrated, angry, anxious, or happy? Check in with yourself and take your emotional temperature. You want to be aware of your emotions and if they might

affect your choices. Are you reaching for food to deal with an emotion, or are you honoring your hunger? You may already be aware
that you have certain foods you reach for when feeling a certain
emotion. Identifying what you're feeling helps you be awake to the
actions and choices you make in response.

When taking your pre-meal emotional temperature check,
ask yourself:

Am I stressed or overwhelmed?

Am I tired, anxious, angry, bored, or lonely?

*Do I crave a specific food I can't stop thinking about,
such as sweets or salty snack foods?*

*Do I want to eat even though I'm not hungry, or do I still
feel full from the last time I ate?*

Do I feel guilty or ashamed for wanting to reach for food?

Conscious Cravings: What Do You Want to Eat?

Write down what you want to eat. Are you craving a doughnut or a
steak? One client recounted a time she really wanted a salad, but
the only option available was a doughnut, so she ate the doughnut,
because she was stuck and hungry. Another client shared about a
time she felt really hot and craved something cool. Because she
was not feeling stressed, she ate two Good Humor Strawberry
Shortcake ice cream bars for dinner. And you know what? She
said they tasted fantastic, because she had honored her craving
and the ice cream bars were physically and psychologically satisfying. She had not been eating to fill an emotional need, rather she
had listened to herself in the moment and responded intuitively.

This is one example of how you can distinguish between a
craving for certain foods versus emotional eating. Assess your

emotions first by checking in with yourself. Next, put the internal judge in silent mode to see what choice you really want to make and why. Instead of automatically choosing the "should" answer in your brain, ask yourself what you want, and consider giving yourself permission to do so. There is nothing more satisfying than honoring your inner voice. It never steers you wrong. The empowerment you feel when you listen to yourself allows you to meet your needs on a higher level.

Conscious Choices: What Did You Eat?

List what food choice you made and compare it with what you wanted to eat. Did it match up? Did you make a different choice? Why? Did your internal judge hijack the conversation and over-rule what you really wanted to eat? How did your environment come into play? Maybe you were craving a big, crunchy salad, but the only option was a bag of chips from the vending machine. Did your emotions take over and you made the food choice you always do? If so, that's OK. Even being aware of why you make certain choices is progress. Small changes add up to big changes as long as you keep trying.

As you get started, you may feel as overwhelmed as if you were chipping away at an iceberg with a spoon. Remember that you're chipping away at what is not needed in order to free yourself up to learn how to listen to yourself again. Lasting change is not an easy or quick process. Give yourself the gift of patience and time so you can reveal your true self.

Goldilocks Guidelines: Portions Just Right for You

When you're trying to make a change in your relationship with food, you might want to record how much you're eating by estimating your portions using hand sizes or even weighing and measuring your food. Recording this level of information can be helpful if it's something you've never considered before. I compare it to spending money. Maybe you've been trying to make what you consider thoughtful choices, but you're still over budget. Sometimes knowing your budget and seeing the calories, or "price tag," on foods lets you understand how much of an investment those foods require. However, if you find that doing so leaves you more stressed or starting to obsess, then skip this step.

The purpose of a food journal is to help you establish a practice of mindful awareness, not to create shame or guilt. It is not for you to judge how much you ate but to be aware, observe, and analyze it like a scientist. The journal is a way to capture information for you to study why you make certain choices and then reflect on that information to better understand your internal motivations and, if necessary, tweak your choices the next time.

Another way to assess your portions is to use the Goldilocks Guidelines. The fairy tale *Goldilocks and the Three Bears* tells the story of a girl who goes walking in the woods and comes upon a house. After knocking on the door and receiving no response, Goldilocks walks in and starts making herself at home. She finds three bowls of porridge on the kitchen table and starts tasting them. The first bowl is too hot, and the second bowl is too cold, but the third bowl is just right, and she happily eats it up until satisfied.

Compare your portions to the Goldilocks Guidelines: Were they not enough, too much, or just right? Ask yourself:

Did I enjoy what I was eating?

Did I continue to eat even though I wasn't really tasting the food anymore?

How fast did I eat? Should I have been awarded the gold medal in speed eating?

Did I eat with a mindset of eating as much as possible?

Did I eat with a mindset of restriction and listening to what my brain was telling me versus what my body wanted?

Did I eat a portion that filled me up just right such that I felt physically satisfied?

Does Your Cup Overfloweth? Assess Your Fullness after Eating

Using the same scale as before, rate your fullness on a scale of 1–10, with 4–5 still being hungry and 10 feeling "holiday meal" full. Ideally, pause your eating around 7–8, where you feel comfortably full or satisfied—where you feel you might need a snack in another three hours or a meal in another six to seven hours. Stop at a point where you feel "even"—not hungry and not too full. You have probably experienced that sensation about 20 minutes after eating, where you feel a little too full and find yourself thinking: *Ugh, those last three to four bites made my tank spill over a bit.*

Many people I work with are often unsure whether or not they feel full and satisfied after eating. On paper, it seems easy to rate fullness, but it is more challenging in practice. If you're unsure if you're still hungry, I recommend pausing and waiting 30 minutes before eating more. A helpful mantra I recommend is to say, "I can always eat." Reminding yourself that food is available, and you have permission to eat later helps reduce anxiety that might come from fear of feeling deprived.

When determining your fullness after eating, ask yourself:

Is my stomach satisfied?

Am I content?

Does food still sound good?

Does my stomach feel overly stuffed?

Years ago, I used to eat at an Asian-inspired vegetarian restaurant at least once a week. One of my favorite dishes was Curry Supreme; it had chunks of vegetarian "chicken" with stewed potatoes, carrots, broccoli, and green peas in a Japanese curry sauce. The portions were huge, and I used to eat the whole thing and feel uncomfortably stuffed, which detracted from the pleasure of eating there. So I devised a strategy whereby I would divide my plate in half and only eat half the total portion when I was at the restaurant and bring the rest home. I told myself that if I was still hungry when I got home, I could eat the rest of the meal. The ride home was about 30 minutes, so it gave me time to digest the food and assess the situation. Sometimes I would go home and still feel satisfied, excited about eating the leftovers the next day for lunch. Other times I would realize I was still physically hungry and would eat the rest of my dinner right away. Practicing this strategy wasn't easy, but with time it became a sustainable habit.

Working on becoming aware of how full you feel after a meal makes you more attuned to the point where you feel comfortable, so that you can pause your eating at that point.

Self-Satisfaction Survey

Record your emotions and satisfaction after eating and compare them to before you started eating. As you think about how you feel, ask yourself:

Do I feel satisfied, frustrated, stressed, or happy?

How did I feel before eating, during eating, and now after eating?

Did I feel content, or did I end up eating other foods in the kitchen before going back to the food I originally wanted?

Did I keep eating even though I didn't feel hungry?

Did I make a food choice that honored what I really wanted to eat, or did I choose a food based on what I thought I should eat?

Journaling helps us be more aware and assess how we are feeling both physically and mentally. Pausing and reflecting on both of these aspects before and after we eat lets us learn more about ourselves and how we react to different factors. Journaling allows us to acknowledge that it's OK to not be OK and to recognize what our emotional triggers are. It helps us to separate hunger cues from emotional cues and to analyze our eating patterns. It can also help us become more comfortable with being uncomfortable and to learn to embrace or sit with negative emotions or feelings rather than using food to run away from internal stress.

It's Alive: Emotions as People

One way to help separate yourself from negative emotions is to think of or describe emotions as people. A 2019 study in the *Journal of Consumer Psychology* (Fangyuan Chen 2019) looked at how thinking of emotions as people changed consumer behavior. Researchers were inspired by the Pixar movie *Inside Out*, in which emotions (joy, sadness, fear, disgust, anger) are seen as cartoonish figures that live inside the young brain of the main character's head and fight for dominance over a board in a master control room. The researchers theorized that making emotions into people would allow participants to detach from feeling sad and increase the chance of making better buying decisions.

In the study, the participants were asked to think of a time they felt sad, such as after the death of someone close. One group wrote about this emotion as if it were a real-life person, while the other group detailed how the emotion affected them. The group that made sadness into people used depictions such as "a little girl walking slowly with her head down," "a pale person with no smile," or "someone with gray hair and sunken eyes." This group rated their sadness on a lower level. The researchers then tested how this affected behavior and self-control. They asked participants in both groups to select either cheesecake or salad as a lunch side dish. The group that rated emotions as people were more likely to choose the healthy salad option. According to study author Li Yang of the University of Texas at Austin, this technique "may be a new way to regulate this emotion. Activating this mindset is a way to help people feel better and resist temptations that may not benefit them in the long term."

To apply this theory in day-to-day life, let's say I'm feeling anxious and all I can think about is munching on a bag of salty chips. Instead of heading straight to the kitchen cupboard, I pause, sit down, and think about how my anxiety would look as a person. I picture a woman like me, with brown hair pulled back in a messy ponytail and frizzy pieces sticking up around her forehead. Let's call her Amy Anxious. Amy has a furrowed brow, and she's sitting on the couch, hugging her bent knees. Her left hand is clutched in a fist placed in front of her mouth, cradling her chin. She has a soft blanket wrapped around her that she's holding tight around her shoulders with her right hand. Her head is pointed down, and she's trying to make herself as compact as possible. I imagine that Amy is a friend and that I want to help her feel better. I visualize maybe gently stroking her hair and telling her, "It's OK." I encourage her to take deep breaths and feel myself slowly breathing in and out as well as I mentally coach her. Suddenly, I realize I'm not craving the chips anymore. I feel more centered and can go on with my day. If I start to feel the anxiety rising, I picture Amy and visualize saying and doing things that would comfort her, rather than relying on food to fix what I'm feeling.

We can use this visualization to manage any emotion, from anxiety to anger.

Sugar-Free Self-Soothing

Another strategy to help manage emotional eating is to identify ways that don't involve food to soothe yourself or provide comfort. Examples include taking a walk, sitting quietly and looking at the clouds, listening to music, taking a drive with the windows down, buying flowers, snuggling in a weighted blanket, lighting a scented candle or incense, taking a bath, listening to the sounds of a small desktop water fountain, watching a funny video or show, reading a book, practicing deep breathing, playing with your dog, knitting, or gardening. Identify as many ways as possible to help manage different feelings. It's like collecting tools in a toolbox, so you can select the best tool for each job. Learning to self-soothe without food is key to forming a healthier relationship with it. Food then becomes more about nourishing your body in a mindful way than a Band-Aid for negative feelings.

Emotional Shapewear

> *Surround yourself with the dreamers and the doers,*
> *the believers and the thinkers, but most of all, surround*
> *yourself with those who see the greatness within you,*
> *even when you don't see it yourself.*
> — Edmund Lee

While social media has provided many ways to connect with others, it can actually increase a sense of aloneness and depression

when people try to hide the harsh reality of life beneath orches-
trated images of perfection. People tend to share only their best
moments of their lives online. While we understand this and
rationally know that creating these images requires a lot of effort,
it can still be challenging to fight that nagging feeling that everyone else's life is great and that you're the only one struggling,
especially with eating.

After the Fourth of July holiday one year, I was talking with
a client who was feeling down as she was alone and inundated by
pictures on social media of her friends and their families enjoying
picnics and celebrations. I reminded her that people tend to show
only the most sanitized version of themselves on social media and
that their composite reality is usually very different. I shared with
her that my Fourth of July holiday involved buying toilet paper
at Target. In our minds, we think everyone is living only the fun,
glamorous life shown in the pictures they post. Most of us, however, are spending our time doing "adulting" chores.

To fight such feelings of isolation and have something to look
forward to beyond a trip to Target to buy toilet paper, it's important to build a social support system. You want to have a network
of family, friends, acquaintances, and counselors or therapists
that make you feel connected and can give you emotional support
when you're dealing with issues that can become overwhelming.
Identify people in your corner who don't judge or criticize you.
Find people who make you feel positive about yourself, listen
to you, provide feedback that is not self-serving, and make you
feel heard. You may talk to them frequently or occasionally. The
support may range from intense conversations about deep personal issues with close friends to fun chats with someone you
stand next to in your exercise class. Your support network can be
anyone in your community who you have occasional or frequent
interactions with who are positive and make you feel happy and
good about yourself. For example, a receptionist in my apartment

building is so friendly, positive, and thoughtful that just talking to her for even a few minutes makes me happy.

Connecting with others in a variety of degrees helps support positive emotional health and, in turn, helps you to cope and be more resilient. Having personal connections allows you to turn to other people for love, kindness, the feeling of belonging, and the knowledge that you matter. You may love food, but food can't love you back. No matter how much or what you eat, it will never fill the emotional void that a connection with others can.

It can be helpful to sit down and brainstorm a list of all the people you have available to create your emotional support network, along with places or situations where you could cultivate that network. Here's a sample list:

- People—family, friends, significant others, coworkers, exercise buddies, neighbors, doctors, dietitians, therapists
- Situations—home, work, school, gyms, exercise class, playing sports, volunteering, church

If your emotional support network needs strengthening, you can use this list to enhance your circle.

Your Environment: Triggering or Supportive?

Another aspect of healthy eating is setting up your environment for success. You can do this by arranging your home and workspace so it's easy to make decisions that support your goals. For example, many people have "trigger foods" that are hard for them to stop eating once they take the first bite. These foods—such as chips, cookies, candy, ice cream, fast food, and soda—tend to be easy to eat and often require a large portion in order to provide satisfaction. My Krispy Kreme binge (described earlier) is a prime example of the power of trigger foods. I recommend that when you're emotionally vulnerable, you take a break from these foods, and if possible, keep them out of the house while you work on stabilizing your emotional foundation.

If living with other people in your household makes it difficult to remove all the foods that might trigger you, another strategy is to look at how your kitchen is set up. Rearrange your shelves and cupboards so any foods you're tempted to grab and start mindlessly munching on are not at eye level. Put them in a higher or lower cupboard that makes the items difficult to reach. One client purchased solid-colored plastic bins to move a family member's snack foods into that person's bedroom. If that's not an option for you, another suggestion is to buy things you don't like, such as a flavor of ice cream or cookies you don't particularly care for. That way you will at least be less interested in eating those items.

Look at what's sitting on your counter and in your cupboards. Once I went to a party where they handed out meringue cookies to take home. I didn't particularly like them, but I left them sitting on my kitchen counter. Every time I walked past the kitchen, I would mindlessly take a little nibble just because I saw them there. I finally pitched them when I woke up to what I was doing. The question I asked myself is, *Would I be even thinking about eating this food choice if I didn't have it at home?* The answer was no. That's why it's important to stock our kitchen with healthy options we like so it's easier to make better choices. It's important that we remember to be very choosy about what we bring into our environment, because if it's in our space, there's a pretty good chance we're going to eat it.

Another factor that can help manage your eating is decluttering your house. According to organizational expert Peter Walsh (2008) in his book *Does This Clutter Make My Butt Look Fat?*, decluttering your house can be the first step to losing weight. Why? Because disorganization can lead to stress, which increases the hormone cortisol as well as blood sugar, which, in turn, increases insulin, making you feel hungrier. For example, if your dining room table and kitchen is piled high with stuff, you're not creating an environment conducive to healthful eating. If you have trouble cooking in your kitchen, finding space in your refrigerator, or don't have a place to sit down and enjoy a meal, isn't it more tempting to eat out and reach for less healthy fast food or grab-and-go items? Packing our homes with "stuff" becomes a symbol of how we might be approaching eating—where more is always better. Yet just like homes cluttered with things we never use, our bodies become storage units for the extra fuel we don't need.

Remember . . . You Have the Power

Danowski reminds her readers that "food doesn't speak and that even if it did, you don't have to listen. You can choose to walk away instead" (Danowski 2007, 16). Cultivating self-awareness of our emotions and patterns in order to change our eating habits is not easy. Like learning an instrument or new language, it feels awkward at first, but the more you practice, the more fluid and automatic it becomes. You have the power.

CHAPTER 13

HUGGING PORCUPINES AND CREATING YOUR EMOTIONAL TOOLBOX

I'm feelin' like a Monday,
but someday I'll be Saturday night.
— Bon Jovi,
from the song "Someday I'll Be Saturday Night"

Creating a healthier relationship with food requires untangling negative thoughts and separating them from your usual habits. It's not easy to recognize and acknowledge negative thought patterns and address the real issues instead of using food as a temporary Band-Aid or distraction. Embracing your feelings rather than running away from them is scary. Our culture tells us to "always look at the positive" or "smile because there's always something to smile about." People ask how you are, and the automatic response is, "I'm good." You fall down as a kid and start to cry, and adults tell you to "walk it off." Modern society and cultural expectations make us believe that it's a badge of honor to be strong and tough when going through difficult times. Sometimes real strength is letting people we trust into our real lives by allowing ourselves to be emotionally vulnerable through expressing how we really feel.

Sometimes life just really sucks. Losing your job, dealing with a pandemic, experiencing a divorce, having a fight with a friend, experiencing money problems, facing the death of a loved one, or falling into health issues are situations many of us have dealt with. It's OK to acknowledge and say that life does suck sometimes rather than talk yourself out of your feelings. To return to the emotional bath fitter image, you don't have to plop a shiny plastic cover over crappy feelings and emotions growing underneath and pretend that your molding soul is just fine. It's OK to admit that you're not OK at times. You're human. We all feel that way.

I tend to think of difficult emotions or times as thunderstorms. You see a storm gathering in the distance, you feel a strange energy in the air, and your antennas pick up a sense of impending doom. As the dark clouds roll in, you hear the thunder, see the lightening, and wait for the rain to let loose. Sometimes during intense storms, the sky becomes so dark the world seems bound to end. It's terrifying, but you keep reminding yourself that you have seen storms before and know this one will be clearing. The sun is on the other side of this; you just need to hold on, you tell yourself.

The more you learn to accept that you will have turbulent times of difficult feelings, the more resilient you will be in the midst of this fact of nature. The more you accept how you are feeling and process it, the sooner the storm subsides and allows you to move in calmer or more settled emotional weather without always relying on food as your umbrella.

NAME INSTEAD OF TAME

To help put food in its proper place, name but don't automatically try and tame or control your emotions. First, acknowledge whether you're angry, lonely, frustrated, tired, happy, sad, or scared. Relaxing through a process where you notice what you're observing, what you're thinking, and how it's making you feel helps to validate what you're feeling. Feelings are authentic, but the stories you tell yourself behind those feelings may or may not be accurate. Thoughts trigger emotions. For example, maybe you're feeling frustrated because you ate too much ice cream and finished the pint even though you were full about halfway through it. The cascade of guilt (feeling bad about the action you took), shame (feeling bad about who you are), and beating yourself up begins as you tell yourself, *I can't believe I did this again. I'm such a failure. I'm never going to lose weight.*

The feelings of fear, frustration, guilt, shame, anxiety, depression, and disappointment are real. However, the story you're telling yourself is not. Making a misstep does not mean you are a failure or are doomed to never achieve your goals. Practice self-compassion and be gentle with yourself in difficult moments by rewriting the script in your head. Instead of saying, *I'm doomed to fail*, acknowledge, *I feel disappointed that I made a choice that wasn't honoring myself or where I want to go, but I can make a different choice the next time.*

Emotions such as disappointment bring us into our present reality to signal us to approach things differently or change our mindset, so we don't get stuck. For example, the disappointment I felt after succumbing to an intense binge episode because I felt so unhappy in my job dumped me into such a miserable physical and emotional low that I became determined I never wanted to feel this way again. At that moment, I decided to embrace my feelings and try to memorize them by filing them in my brain. Later, when I faced difficult moments and wanted to use food to make myself feel better, I would then retrieve these feelings from my mental filing cabinet to remind myself to make a different choice.

HUGGING YOUR PORCUPINES

Allow yourself, as uncomfortable as it can be, to sometimes sit with your emotions instead of running away from them. When dealing with difficult emotions, I tend to think of that old joke:

"How do you hug a porcupine? Very carefully." I visualize difficult emotions as porcupines, and I think, *Embracing them is going to suck, and I might get stuck with some quills, but I'm going to make peace with this animal in order to figure out how to coexist. I may not like it, but I'm not going to fear it.* Instead of shying away from uncomfortable emotions such as anger, shame, anxiety, or grief, practicing being aware of what we're feeling can help us take the next step to understanding what is triggering these emotions.

Letting go of the need to control our emotions frees us up to watch these feelings unfold and organically dissipate rather than having to turn to food to self-medicate. Through practice, we can remind ourselves that difficult emotions are fleeting, and that food provides only a temporary distraction that doesn't address the true issues. Learning to hug your porcupines or lean into them doesn't mean you have to deal with the quills by yourself. I recommended seeking the support of a therapist to help navigate your underlying emotional landscape and understand how it impacts your relationship with food.

> *Thank you so much for bringing up such a painful*
> *subject. While you're at it, why don't you give me*
> *a nice paper cut and pour lemon juice on it?*
> — Inigo Montoya,
> character in the movie *The Princess Bride*

SELF-CARE STRATEGIES: YOUR EMOTIONAL TOOLBOX

While you're working on creating space between thoughts and feelings, it is important to identify and use techniques that will help you deal with your emotions without using food to do so. In this section, we're going to explore some ideas and techniques for you to incorporate toward this end.

First, Create and Fill Your Emotional Toolbox

To create a useful emotional toolbox, you have to first fill it with a number of "tools" or activities to take the place of using food to soothe or distract yourself. Identifying a list of activities ahead of time—when you're not in a vulnerable state and feeling overwhelmed or stressed—allows you to select the right tool for the job at hand rather than having to think about creating such a tool in the moment. When you're feeling unsettled, a predetermined plan of action is the easiest kind to implement.

A good self-soothing kit will include a variety of tools that employ all our senses of sight, smell, taste, touch, and sound to help keep us grounded. Years ago, I found a dumb joke book in a bookstore that made me laugh so hard even though it was filled with "dad jokes." The book still helps me feel joy, even in a dark time. Music can also be helpful. You might have certain songs, for example, that open your internal release valve, giving you permission to remove the lock from the teary floodgates and experience sweet release. Sounds of nature, the ocean, or waterfalls can also be soothing. Taking a bath, simmering cinnamon and spices on the stove, or wrapping yourself in a favorite sweater are other sensory ways to instill calm. For me, wearing cute dog slippers provides physical comfort for my feet and makes me smile every time I see the creatures' happy faces. Watching a show or video, reading a book, or calling a friend can also help provide time to process your feelings instead of using food for comfort. I drink Japanese green tea, since the process of brewing it calms my mind and the warm liquid comforts me. One client who struggled with overeating in social situations began carrying a smooth "worry" stone in her pocket, so that when she reached in and held it in her hand, it reminded her of her intention to pause before taking second helpings.

In addition to soothing activities, identify purposeful, distracting activities, tasks, or chores to let out some of the stressful energy. Puzzles, books, and games can be both soothing and distracting activities. If you're feeling stressed, bored, or anxious, or you're feeling OK but just fighting the urge to snack, engage in a task that helps you accomplish something that needs to get done. For example, you may want to take a walk, vacuum the house, pay some bills, or go and do an errand to get yourself out of the house. Some clients take up knitting since it keeps their hands busy and distracts them from snacking. Personally, I've set about organizing drawers and cleaning out closets, since I tend to get lost in that task and forget about snacking. Getting involved in purposeful tasks often makes you feel better by accomplishing something that needed to get done while at the same time preventing you from eating for the sake of eating when you are not hungry.

Calming Countdown

Another strategy I've suggested to clients is called the 5-4-3-2-1 technique. This is actually a technique to help deal with anxiety, but it can be used any time you feel your emotions or thoughts are spiraling up and you need to re-ground yourself before mindlessly reaching for food.

You can use the calming countdown when you're feeling so overwhelmed by your emotions that you can't even think of what tool to select from your emotional toolbox.

Here are the five steps:

5 – Acknowledge FIVE things you see around you, such as papers sitting on your desk, a picture on the wall, or anything in your surroundings.

4 – Acknowledge FOUR things you can touch around you, such as the arm of the chair you're sitting in, the back of your neck, or your feet on the carpet.

3 – Acknowledge THREE things you hear. Focus on any sound external to your body, such as a bird chirping outside your window, the sound of the garbage truck rolling down the street, or the sound of the laundry whirling in the dryer.

2 – Acknowledge TWO things you can smell, such as the scent of laundry soap woven into a freshly washed t-shirt, or maybe the smell of a wood-burning stove as you walk in your neighborhood during the fall.

1 – Acknowledge ONE thing you can taste. What does the inside of your mouth taste like? Gum, coffee, or the sandwich from lunch?

Taking deep breaths while going through this calming exercise will help bring you into the present moment and resettle you. It will give you a way to separate your thoughts from your emotions by temporarily focusing on tangible things in your environment.

Your emotional toolbox is a learning process that requires you to find out what works for you. For example, I find intense exercise very stress relieving while another person might find gentle yoga to be the respite they need. One person might love to listen to the sounds of the rain forest while another person might find listening to heavy-metal music at an ear-piercing volume in their car to be the perfect remedy. Not every tool will be a match for every person or situation, so it's important to reflect without judgment on what works for you. Learning what coping skills/tools are helpful for you fosters an intuitive and mindful perspective.

WHEN AND HOW TO USE YOUR EMOTIONAL TOOLBOX

The next step is learning when and how to use your emotional toolbox. Because this step is not always intuitive with your new tools, let's look at some familiar scenarios. Imagine you're at work, for example, and you're feeling pressured to complete a project.

The stress feels overwhelming, and all you can think about is visiting the vending machine and punching the button for a candy bar. It feels like the only bright spot on a difficult day. Imagine also that you just ate lunch and know you're not really hungry, but food is all you can think about. Pause and try to identify what you're really feeling. You determine that you're stressed, not hungry, and really need to take a break for a few minutes to help reset your emotional compass. It's not about the food. It's about allowing yourself some breathing space. You realize you don't need the excuse of the candy bar to stop and pause. So instead, you decide to walk around the block a few times while listening to music to help relieve some of the pressure.

Now imagine you're at home and you just had a fight with your significant other or your kids. They just pushed your hot button, sending your mood from managing to mad. Very mad. You need an escape, and you head to the kitchen, throw open the freezer door, and grab the half gallon of ice cream. You whip a spoon out of the drawer, plunge it into the ice cream like a mini shovel, and lift it to your mouth. In quick, successive digs you continue excavating. You're not even tasting the ice cream, and you're still angry. Suddenly, you remember your toolbox. You throw the spoon in the sink, place the ice cream back in the freezer, and pause. As the heat pulsates off your cheeks, you close your eyes and take a few deep breaths. You start becoming aware of how the anger is showing up in your body as you feel the tension in your neck and the possible start of a headache. You keep breathing and start the calming countdown—five things you can see, four things you can touch, three things you can hear, two things you can smell, and one thing you can taste . . . the lingering remains of ice cream. You think that no matter how much ice cream you eat, it's only a temporary distraction and it's not addressing the real issue. Eating the ice cream to soothe your emotions is only contributing to another problem—managing your weight. As you continue to breathe, you start feeling some of the anger dissipate. Some of the tension in your body eases, and you decide to go do an errand and call your friend on the way to talk through what you're feeling. You realize it's not about the ice cream. It's about being heard and supported and knowing that you and your feelings matter.

SUPPORTIVE ENVIRONMENT

While all foods can fit into a balanced diet, I usually recommend removing trigger foods from your environment while you're working on your strategies to address emotional eating. Taking a break from them while you get more settled often helps relieve some of the stress and pressure when those foods are not in arm's reach. Their absence forces you to pause and think about why you are craving them, rather than automatically eating them and wondering after the fact what the driving reason was.

As I was working on healing my own relationship with food, I took a break from buying ice cream to help provide space from the ability to automatically grab and eat it when the urge hit. I told myself I could eat ice cream but I would need to go to Dairy Queen or McDonald's and buy an ice cream cone or small sundae to help manage becoming overwhelmed by wanting to eat large portions. As I mentally acclimated to the idea that I could eat ice cream every day if I wanted to, suddenly the permission to eat this food made it not such a big deal anymore. Ice cream became just another food that I was able to transition to, including in my freezer, without feeling the need to eat it all at once.

Have you begun noticing thoughts, understanding the emotions they provoke, and then learning to let those emotions go to allow you to move forward into new emotional territory? Are you working on fully stocking your emotional toolbox to give yourself access to a variety of tools you can select as needed for the job, rather than always reaching for food? If so, these self-created resources will help you begin healing your relationship with food. Hmm . . . I think you might have just started hugging a porcupine.

CHAPTER 14

PRACTICING MINDFULNESS WITHOUT JUDGMENT

*If we suspend judgment and look to how we can make
conscious choices to uplift the situation, we can be sure
that we are doing all we can to attract a happier and
more harmonious outcome.*
—Deepak Chopra

We all have an inner critic who makes judgments about everything in life. From the time we get up in the morning until we go to sleep at night, our inner voice yaps constantly. Some mornings when I look in the mirror, my inner voice starts talking and trying to set the tone for the day: *Uh, Mary, you look tired and worn out. Is that a gray hair I see? I think you need to do some more ab work. Girl, you need to get it together.* Just typing this, I feel myself shrinking and hunching over because, unfortunately, this conversation is more familiar than I would like to admit.

Often these internal, judgmental conversations lead to negative thoughts quickly multiplying and spiraling out of control about other areas of our life. *Ugh, I look so bad this morning. I feel like such a failure. Why didn't Sheila text me back yet? Did I say something wrong? Oh no, she's probably mad at me. I never say anything right. Wait, is that dust? This house is a mess. My life is spinning out of control. I'm going to die with bad hair, friendless, and alone in a messy apartment. What is wrong with me?*

When we start sliding down the rabbit hole and being swallowed up into mental darkness, we might think that judging ourselves harshly will snap us into action, that being hard on ourselves will spark a self-control that we haven't yet been able to achieve, that negativity will be the answer to solving the things we aren't happy with. Has being hard on ourselves ever worked as a long-term solution? Yeah, not so much.

Our internal critic does not hesitate to offer its strong opinions when it comes to food. It might employ a judge and jury that pronounces us "good" for eating perceived healthy foods and "bad" for eating what we consider unhealthy or more processed foods. Guilt and shame accompany these sentences, and we might start following strict rules to try to scare ourselves into not committing these dieting "crimes" again.

DIET DECEPTION

I hear many prevalent dieting rules from the clients I work with. Popular dieting culture has us convinced that if we're "good" and do what we're told, these rules will magically guarantee our success. These types of diets rules are examples of a cognitive distortion or "stinking thinking" called Heaven's Reward Fallacy. The falsehood is that if we follow the rules, we can start magically "expecting all sacrifice and self-denial to pay off, as if there were someone keeping score. We will then feel disappointed and even bitter when the reward does not come" (Substance Abuse and Mental Health Services Administration 2012).

Common diet rules I typically hear are:

Don't eat past 8 p.m.; your body stores everything as fat.

Avoid bread; bread is a weight-loss devil.

Fruit is bad and has too much sugar.

Don't eat anything white—white pasta, white rice, white bread, potatoes.

Never skip breakfast.

Never eat breakfast; you should be fasting.

The problem with these types of rules is that they reinforce binary thinking, or what I call the "light-switch mentality" that we talked about earlier, where you're either "right or wrong" or "on or off," classifying everything as all or nothing. With this way of looking at things, you feel deprivation is your ticket to salvation. The problem is, you make one misstep and violate these rules and you feel everything is ruined. It's like getting a scratch on your car and deciding to compound the whole vehicle—*I'll just push it off this cliff and start over.*

This mentality makes getting started harder, as you often won't get refocused or work on things again until you have an imaginary clean slate. For example, maybe you haven't been exercising because your schedule has been very busy. Instead of thinking, *Maybe I can fit in 10–15 minutes of walking now*, you tell yourself, *Well, I'll wait until Monday to start* . . . but today is only Tuesday. Instead of eating a few cookies, you end up eating the entire package because you feel you've "blown it," and you start bargaining with yourself about never eating these cookies ever again.

NO SHAME, NO BLAME: BE YOUR OWN BEST FRIEND

OK, so how do you start taking action if shame and blame are no longer your ride-or-die friends?

The first step is to clear out the noise of your inner voice by challenging what it's telling you. To do this, you begin by creating separation between your thoughts and your feelings. You then make observations as you become aware of your inner conversation, and you extend grace, compassion, empathy, and understanding to yourself rather than judgement. Pretend you are talking to your close friend. What would you say to them?

Let's take my earlier example of my thoughts spiraling out of control in a leap from being critical of my appearance to Sheila hating me and then dying alone in a dusty apartment. Rewriting the script—in the presence of observation, empathy, and compassion—might sound like this: *Wow, Mary, you look tired this morning. You've been working so hard and not getting enough rest. Sheila must be just as busy because I haven't heard back from her. My apartment is dusty, but I've been too busy to clean. The dust will wait for me, so I think I will do something fun this weekend to give myself a break from my intense schedule. Maybe I will make an appointment to get my hair done, since that is always a treat and makes me feel relaxed and pampered.*

Rewriting the script allows us to be more of a supporter, moderator, or reconciler than a judge or jury. Life is hard enough; we don't need to make it any harder on ourselves.

Taking this same approach, let's examine some of those "diet rules" you might have imposed on yourself, then identify the distortion in them and see how you can question your inner critic and view things differently.

DEBUNK DIET MYTHS

Don't eat past 8 p.m.; your body stores everything as fat.

Instead of telling yourself, *Don't eat past 8 p.m.*, question this belief. Ask yourself, *So does that mean that I don't store body fat at 7:59 p.m. but suddenly at 8 p.m. I become a fat-storage machine?* I don't think so. Whether your weight increases or decreases is based on what you do over extended periods of time, such as days and weeks. Think of energy balance like a bank account with income and expenses. If you're eating more energy or taking in more calorie income than you're burning off or spending, your weight (or your bank balance) will increase. If you're eating less than you're burning off and are in a calorie deficit (less calorie income), your weight (or bank balance) will decrease.

Instead of identifying a magical time to stop eating, rewrite the script and think about a guideline where you check in with yourself in the evening and ask, *Am I really physically hungry or just emotionally hungry? Am I bored, tired, restless, or stressed?* A good indication that you're experiencing emotional or "head hunger" is when you find yourself searching the kitchen and opening the refrigerator and cupboards while thinking, *I want something, but I don't know what I want.* Sometimes emotional hunger manifests as a craving for a specific food, such as cookies or ice cream. Physical hunger has bodily cues of a rumbling stomach and difficulty concentrating and can be satisfied by many different food choices. One strategy is to ask yourself, *Am I hungry enough to eat an apple?* If the answer is no, you might be dealing with "head" hunger.

Avoid bread, fruit, and anything white—white pasta, white rice, white bread, potatoes.

Let's look at the concept of avoiding bread, fruit, or any "white" carb such as rice, pasta, or potatoes. I always like to joke that no one ever came to see me or had health problems because they ate one too many bananas. When Oprah invested in Weight Watchers and did a commercial where she said she could now eat bread, a slew of clients came knocking on my door both amazed and livid—amazed that Oprah was eating bread and losing weight and livid that for years they had been hearing the opposite message, that forbidding bread was an essential part of losing weight.

To repeat, in terms of managing your weight, what matters is not one food but matching up your movement patterns with how much you're eating based on your goals. Healthy eating means eating a variety of foods that you enjoy and that nourish your body and support your health.

Question your inner critic about whether one food is the devil and is causing all your issues. One food or meal doesn't make you healthy, and one food or meal doesn't make you unhealthy. Reflect on whether there is an imbalance in your variety of food choices and whether you're eating one food or type of food so much that it's crowding out other choices. Ask yourself if your eating patterns are beneficial or harmful to your physical and emotional health.

Never skip breakfast versus never eat breakfast.

Regarding the diametrically opposed rules of a) always eat breakfast versus b) never eat breakfast, ask yourself, *Am I hungry in the morning?* I work with some people for whom breakfast is their favorite meal and with others who can't stand the thought of food first thing in the morning. Consider when you are naturally hungry. If you like eating a bigger lunch or dinner, then honor that natural hunger pattern. If you look forward to breakfast in the morning, then fasting until later in the day is probably not a strategy you want to employ. Since we can find research that supports either approach, the most important factor is taking into account your lifestyle and preferences.

Trusting and listening to yourself leads to more mindful, intuitive eating as you make food choices based on hunger and fullness levels, satisfaction, and how food makes you feel, rather than what you "should" do. Don't be afraid to listen to yourself. You are your own best expert and usually already know the answer to what works for you.

CHAPTER 15

MOVING FORWARD

Growth is painful. Change is painful. But nothing is as painful as staying stuck somewhere you don't belong.
— Mandy Hale

LOVE WRAPPED IN FUR

In my early 20s, as I was settling into my first career working for the federal government, I embarked on a search for my first dog as an adult. I scoured the animal shelters and other dog rescues, eyes peeled for a match. At the time, I lived in the Washington, DC, suburbs, where I found Friends of Homeless Animals, a rescue organization. My parents happened to be visiting on a beautiful fall October weekend, and we drove to the shelter almost an hour away. It was packed to capacity, with two dogs per cage. My mom and I peered through each cage and talked to each animal, looking for a connection. I walked several dogs and was about to give up hope that I would find a match that day when my mom called me over to one of the cages.

In the cage in front of her was a small white dog, about 30 pounds. A terrier mix, she could have been the dog Toto from *The Wizard of Oz*, except she was white with much larger, pointier ears. As my mom spoke to her, she moved her head from side to side, all the while staring at my mother's face as though thoughtfully taking in everything being said. As the conversation continued, one of the dog's ears adorably flopped over. We asked to walk her, and I immediately felt a connection. The shelter didn't know anything about the dog's background, except that she had been found abandoned on a rural road. While knowing her history would have been nice, it didn't matter to me. I already had the most important information I needed—that this dog was desperate to be loved and cared for and that my heart had already fallen for her that day.

The shelter had given my new companion the name Baby, but I renamed her Tilly, short for Chantilly in honor of the place near where she was found. Tilly quickly became my shadow, always by my side. As a rescue dog, Tilly needed about a year of consistent care to become healthy and settled, but the emotional scars of her unknown past trauma showed up in unusual ways, much the way our past traumas can affect our relationship with food. Untreated and unresolved traumas can show up as disordered eating patterns. Bingeing can be a way to try and fill an emotional void, while purging can be a way to try and get rid of unpleasant memories (Coker Ross 2017).

A few months after I adopted Tilly, it was close to Christmas and I had wrapped up a package of gourmet dog cookies and placed them under the Christmas tree. I was living in a small ground-floor apartment at the time and had gone out to dinner. When I returned home and opened the door, I immediately saw brightly colored holiday wrapping paper ripped apart and strewn across the living room floor along with the empty container that had housed the dog cookies. Without warning, Tilly bolted out of the open door and flew into the apartment complex neighborhood. Stunned, I tried to process the scene, then turned and ran down the street, desperately calling, "Tillie! Tillllieee!" But the streets remained quiet except for one man walking his dog. Anguished, I asked if he had seen her, letting myself hope for a moment.

"No, I haven't," he said. My heart fell. After continuing to call Tillie and combing the neighborhood, I finally made my way back toward my apartment with a downcast heart. Who should be waiting at the door but my beautiful, sweet Tilly, seemingly smiling at me like nothing was wrong. Whatever past trauma Tilly had endured had caused her to assume that I would be furious about her getting into her Christmas present and eating all the cookies. In her mind, running away was safer than the punishment she assumed was coming.

Tilly's emotions were real, but her assumptions about how I would react were unfounded. I knew I would love and cherish my precious Tilly and help her feel settled, and after her automatic reaction from past trauma subsided, she was able to let go and find her way back to me. She knew in her heart I would be there for her.

Although Tilly is an animal, we see this tendency to react to current situations based on previous experiences in humans as well. Past trauma impacts us, which, in turn, impacts our relationship with food. Tillie's story shows that no matter what we've been through, however, no matter how difficult our journey has been, a glimmer of hope still resides in us. Many of my clients who've struggled their whole lives with their relationship with food often express skepticism that "this time" will be different. I know how hard it is for someone to walk through my door and open themself up to ask for help. But the fact that they have the courage to show up demonstrates that they still have hope and believe things can be different. And the fact that you have the courage and openness to read this book shows the same for you.

THE ZEN OF DOGS

Animals, especially dogs, can show us different ways to deal with and approach challenges in our life. Just by being themselves, dogs remind us of the importance of being nurtured, showing us that we, too, can overcome past emotional damage. Tilly was able to overcome her fear in the moment by holding onto the promise of love. She had picked me for a reason, and rather than run away never to be found, she faced her own insecurities and came back to me. She wanted to move forward. I know we want to move forward, too, so we can learn how to start healing our disruptive eating patterns and finally trust that we have the knowledge and skills to truly nourish ourselves without stress or judgement. Animals teach us how to focus on living in the moment rather than getting bogged down in the past.

GETTING UNSTUCK

If we are desperate to move forward, why is there a disconnect between what we want and what we actually do? How do we get unstuck and pry ourselves free from the hamster wheel of habits that has brought us here in the first place? In our hearts, we're desperate for change, but something unseen seems to be holding us back from moving into that change.

I've worked with many clients who have struggled with feeling stuck. Years ago, I worked with a client who had her own catering company, two gym memberships, and a personal trainer. Her catering company would make her any food she asked them to. The trainer would come to her house. On paper, she had every advantage that many people dream of and think, *If I only had this, I could be successful.* However, this particular client didn't lose weight. She was stuck, not by her circumstances, but by her mindset. Rationally she knew she needed to change, but mentally she was not ready for it. To move forward, we must accept and embrace a new way of doing things. It can be very scary and uncomfortable to do something a different way.

For many years, I felt stuck in my job. It wasn't until my disordered eating patterns made me so miserable that I finally realized I was experiencing symptoms of my unhappiness. My body and mind were trying to tell me that things needed to change. It took me 10 years to finally listen deeply enough to pull the trigger and go back to school.

We're often hesitant to change, because familiarity is calming and makes us feel secure. Take, for example, a small change such as eating with chopsticks. If you've been used to eating with a fork and have never used chopsticks before, you will likely feel awkward and uncomfortable at first. You'll probably eat a lot slower and with less precision, spilling a little food on the table or on yourself. You may feel frustrated that eating is not as easy as it used to be, and think, *Why am I doing this?* But if you continue to practice, it becomes easier and easier and you don't have to concentrate on the new fine motor skills as intensely.

The way we tackle the big changes is actually through a multi-step process that we will explore in the next section.

SIX STAGES OF CHANGE

Changing your habits is challenging and requires persistent effort and a gradual progression of small steps toward your goal. Sometimes you may not understand why you're feeling stuck and having a hard time moving forward. When we break down how change happens, it actually involves a complex six-step process (Snetselaar 2004). Understanding these six steps can help you recognize where you are in the process and how to work through each stage. In this section, we will explore each stage of change and discuss an exit strategy for each one. Keep in mind that although I've broken change down into steps here, it is a very fluid, organic process and often involves sliding back and forth between stages.

Stage 1: Pre-contemplation—"I See Nothing" or "It's Not My Fault" Stage

During this first "pre-contemplation" phase, you may not even recognize there's a problem. You may not have fully acknowledged the consequences of your choices and therefore are blind to them. You may feel you have no control over your behavior or habits and have given up.

One client, for example, lost weight but then went through a difficult time after his father died, and he regained the weight he had lost. He resumed the habits that had helped him lose weight previously—such as working out, tracking his food intake, and making balanced food choices—but nothing was happening. He became convinced something was wrong with his body because he was doing "everything right." We tested his metabolism and body composition several times, reviewed his food logs, and ordered blood work, specifically looking at his thyroid. Everything was normal. In theory and on paper he should have been losing weight, but he wasn't, and he was frustrated.

One afternoon, we reviewed everything again. I approached our job together as though we were detectives, inspecting every piece of information and determined to crack the case. When we started talking about the weekends, we discovered he was cooking with a lot of oil and not taking that into account. He was also eating out on the weekends and having a few alcoholic drinks but not taking that into consideration either. Plus, he was snacking in the afternoons but not recording those snacks.

Was he purposely trying to be deceitful and hide the truth? Absolutely not. He was just being human. It's like when you get stopped for speeding and the cop asks how fast you were going— you might shave off 5–10 miles. As a human being, because you want to present yourself in the best light both externally and internally, you might tweak or sanitize a story without even realizing you're doing so. You might think, *Well, eating a little bit of this won't matter.* But it does. Your body recognizes how much you're eating and how much you're moving even if part of your brain does not. Denial is a very strong coping mechanism whose purpose is to help you cope with a distressing situation or difficult information until you have time to process whatever came your way.

Challenging denial typically precedes any change in behavior. Denial only becomes a problem when it lingers and prevents you from facing the truth of the consequences of your behavior.

Exit Strategy: Become a Super Sleuth

To move forward through this stage, be like a detective and analyze your behavior. The goal is to raise your self-awareness. Think about your current habits and reflect on them. What steps in your routine are so second nature that you are not accounting for them? Think of all your habits and behavior like money being withdrawn from your checking account. Regardless of whether you spend $100 or $10, it comes out of your bank account. Consistent small withdrawals can add up to a big impact. Consider your habits in the same light. Recognizing there is an issue is the first step to change.

What are you giving yourself a pass on instead of admitting it is probably adding up to a big impact? Have you already tried changing your behavior regarding this? What would be the trigger or "final straw" for you to consider it to be a problem? Are your habits damaging to yourself or others?

Stage 2: Contemplation—Being "On the Fence"

During the contemplation phase, you are able to acknowledge there is a problem. You start thinking about the problem but are not ready to change it. Usually, an indication that someone is in this stage is when they come to see me, saying, "I know what to do, but I'm just not doing it." Somehow you think that having the knowledge means you should be able to put it into action. I always like to joke, "I know how to save money, but I'm still not a millionaire yet." Just because we know something doesn't mean we're ready to act on it. Often you might feel very conflicted because you can see the benefit of making a change but the costs or fear of discomfort of doing something differently are preventing you from moving forward

One client knew that overeating snack foods was an issue for her and was preventing her from reaching her goals. Just thinking of making a change to this habit caused her very high levels of stress and anxiety. She found it terrifying to change the quantities and rituals she was used to, because she considered them almost like friends that she was rejecting. The connection was so strong that she felt a deep sense of loss similar to the death of a loved one even when we just discussed making a change.

Exit Strategy: Fence Post Freedom

To remove the fence post that's holding you back, you need to view change not just as losing something but also as gaining a benefit— such as physical or mental health. Changing your life has to be bigger than a number on the scale. It has to be about the vision of what you want your life to be like and whom you want to be. Having a bigger vision helps you connect with why this change is important to you. It allows you to see the pros and cons of doing something differently and how that plays into what you envision. Identifying what the barriers are to making changes will help you resolve your uncertainty and embrace that this is what you're going to do.

One client, for example, was motivated to lose weight so she would have the energy and mobility to play with her grandkids. Another client was motivated to start walking because she was planning a trip to Europe and wanted to have the stamina to tour everything she wanted without pain. Another client was motivated to change when she saw her blood sugar numbers creeping up and was determined to avoid medication.

When you tie your change to a bigger vision, you have something tangible to hold onto. Instead of thinking, *Ugh I have to walk,* you start thinking, *Walking today is going to help me increase my stamina. If I'm consistent I can see myself walking on my trip and not being distracted or held back by pain.* Small decisions suddenly become connected to a bigger picture, which makes them more meaningful. It's easier to change when you can see how a decision today is going to support a goal or vision of your future self. Your motivation and confidence start to increase as you consistently work on small tasks and start seeing progress. For example, maybe you could only walk for 10 minutes at first, but by walking short distances consistently, you can now easily walk for 30 minutes. Maybe you were drinking a can of soda every day but are now drinking only one a few times a week. As big tasks are broken down into manageable pieces, these mini habits lead to a cycle of success.

Stage 3: Preparation—Laying the Groundwork

In this stage, you're preparing to make the change. You are starting to take responsibility for or ownership of your journey and looking into creating a plan of action. You have graduated from just thinking about making a change and are now committed to action, but you are still considering how to go about it. Your next step is to identify tangible actions you will implement and information or resources you need to make these actions happen.

This stage is similar to preparing for a trip. You've already identified where you want to go (stage 2), and now you're doing the pre-work needed to arrive successfully—you're making travel arrangements and packing your suitcase. In other words, you're collecting information about how to change and start taking small steps to get ready for that journey.

One client who wanted to work on drinking more water bought a large water bottle with times marked on the side to remind her to drink throughout the day. Other clients who wanted to add more movement into their lives bought new exercise clothes so they would have something to wear that they felt good in. And for many clients concerned with making healthy choices when eating out, we've reviewed the menu together in advance to see what they like to eat and to identify strategic choices beforehand.

Exit Strategy: Pack Your Suitcase

Determine your goals and set your plan of action. Start laying the groundwork for how you're going to make changes. For example, for weight loss, you may start making small changes like giving up drinking soda or not buying snack foods after you have eaten what's in your cupboard. You may set up an appointment with a dietitian or decide to join a group weight management program. Maybe you start looking into joining a gym and researching online to see which one might be a fit for your goals. Maybe you want to start drinking more water and, like my client I mentioned, you buy a new water bottle with time markings that remind you to drink a certain amount every few hours. Having the details worked out in advance frees you up to take action rather than spending time wondering what you should do.

Stage 4: Action—Moving the Needle; Matching up Your Actions with Your Intentions

The action phase involves actually "doing it"—taking steps toward change before your habits are fully ingrained or stabilized.

*We are what we repeatedly do. Excellence, then, is not
an act, but a habit and life isn't just a series of events,
but an ongoing process of self-definition.*
— Aristotle

The only way to change your life long term is to change your daily habits. Consistent action must match up with your intention to make true progress. For example, let's pretend you're going on a road trip. In the previous preparation phase, you punched your destination into your GPS; in this action phase, you're listening to the directions and actually driving the car. Think of taking action like moving the needle on the speedometer in your car. You want to apply enough pressure on the pedal so you can see that your car is moving forward but not so much that you're going at an unsafe and unsustainable velocity. Because each person's journey is unique, your speed should be tailored to your comfort level rather than someone else's.

For example, way before I was a dietitian, when I wanted to lose weight, I started with eating a salad at lunch and walking each day. I picked two things I knew I could accomplish and did them consistently. Others choose different goals. One client found her eating journey challenged by snacking in the evening, so she decided to stop eating after dinner.

Exit Strategy: Feed Your Need for Speed

You may be wondering how you can consistently make changes when you feel like you've been struggling for so long.

Changing your life doesn't mean having to change everything at once. In fact, such an approach seldom works; it usually either overwhelms us or burns us out from trying to change too much too soon and, as a result, we rocket back into our previous habits.

It's about aligning our intentions with actions that we can do. When you're in the moment and ready to do your usual habits, stop and ask yourself, *What if I were to make a different choice?* Don't worry about what you did yesterday or what is going to happen tomorrow; just ask, *In this moment, right now, what can I do to help move myself in the direction I want to go?*

Maybe, for example, you've been eating more snack foods than you had intended and feel disappointed that you took that turn in the road. Instead of dwelling on your disappointment, ask yourself, *What can I do right now that will honor the direction I want to move into?* Maybe it's taking a short walk to get a different perspective. Maybe it's choosing a piece of fruit as a snack. I'm a very visual person, so often I "see" my inner negative self-talk as words and phrases floating around outside my head. I sometimes take my hands in front of my eyes and, with my palms facing out, I literally push away my negative thoughts as if they were pesky insects invading my space. Sometimes I even say no aloud or internally to signal to these negative thoughts, *Nope, you're not getting in my head.* This allows me to remove the noise of my own self-doubt and focus on what I can do instead.

Often it would be so easy to say, "forget it" and not do anything at all. Like when I don't have as much time to exercise as I had originally hoped. But then I remind myself, *I have 20 minutes. I can do something in 20 minutes, and that is better than doing nothing.*

Investing energy in past mistakes or deciding you can't do something before you even try is not helpful. Observe and understand why you've made certain choices, but don't let that prevent you from focusing on what you are able to do. Clearing out the noise and being present is one of the most powerful tools we can use. These moments, when strung together consistently, will change your habits and your life. Time always moves quickly. You have a choice every day of how you're going to spend it.

Stage 5: Maintenance—Not Falling Off the Wagon, and "Living It"

During the maintenance phase, you are successfully making changes and are able to keep them up. You're meeting your goals and feeling more confident that the changes you have made are sustainable. If you misstep or detour, you don't let it derail you; you regroup and keep going. Your new habits are feeling more routine, and you don't have to invest as much energy in thinking about them. Like playing an instrument, instead of having to practice each phrase over and over, you have laid a foundation so you can play the entire piece of music and hear the entire song.

One client was struggling to eat on a regular basis. He was busy during the day, didn't bring food with him, and then would either skip meals, eat fast food, or go to the vending machine, since that was his only other available food option. In the evenings, because he hadn't eaten much during the day, he would often eat a large dinner and snack at night. After we worked together to create easy meal and snack ideas with grab-and-go product suggestions, he was able to settle into a regular eating routine. Finding healthy foods he enjoyed that were easy to prepare or assemble allowed him to eat on a consistent basis, since he had planned his meals and snacks. Instead of eating most of his food in the evening, he was able to enjoy a moderate dinner and feel satisfied afterward. His list of go-to meals and snacks were like songs in a playlist that could be easily rotated to keep eating interesting and enjoyable. This made maintaining healthy habits easy because he didn't have to think about new food ideas every day.

Exit Strategy: Self-Care Strong Roots—Your Foundational "Must-Dos"

> Be like a flower, survive the rain but use it to grow.
> — Anonymous

One of the characteristics of dieting is its definite start-and-stop nature. Often a person is willing to undergo more extreme restrictions and diet rules because they know they will only be suffering for a defined period of time. The pitfall of this approach is that if you don't change your lifestyle habits, you end up in the same place—or sometimes even worse—as you slip back into old habits. As you read this, you may be thinking about all the diets you've followed over your lifetime and how each rebound got worse and worse each time you dieted.

Creating some self-care strong roots that become part of your daily routine will help you maintain your new lifestyle. These roots are the behaviors and habits that ground you and help you continue to grow and support your desired changes. Like brushing your teeth or unloading the dishwasher, it's not always a thrill a minute, but you know that if you neglect these things, you start to feel unstable, since you're not watering your foundation. Examples of self-care roots include getting adequate sleep, engaging in movement that you enjoy, practicing deep breathing, carving out alone time, reading, listening to music, engaging in a hobby you enjoy (from gardening to knitting to playing video games). Self-care can include any activity that makes you feel centered, grounded, and nurtured. Ideally you will extend the same level of self-care to yourself that you do for other people.

You need these nonnegotiable foundational habits in your life, where you don't give yourself an "out," because you can always find an excuse—I'm too tired, too busy, too stressed. Letting yourself off the hook only lets you down and becomes a self-fulfilling prophecy.

One of my self-care roots is to get movement every day—whether that be formal exercise, such as running or lifting weights, or informal movement, such as doing some walking errands. For me it's much bigger than physical health; I notice how much movement helps support my mental health as well. Movement helps smooth out my mindset by physically releasing anxious energy, allowing me to focus better the rest of the day. Exercise also gives me a nice endorphin kick. I'm extremely amused internally when I stop at the grocery store after an intense exercise class and my endorphin-infused persona makes me feel like a homecoming queen riding in a Cadillac in the local parade. I just want to smile and wave and say hello to everyone in the produce section. Does that mean I always feel like getting movement in? Nope. Believe me, I spend the first 10 minutes of any run or exercise class questioning my life choice to do this, but I've exercised long enough to know the feeling doesn't last and I will be fine once I get into it and always feel happy that I did it.

Setting your self-care foundational habits eliminates the noise of fighting yourself and debating whether or not you're going to do them. You've already made the decision they're going to happen, so you can focus your energy on taking action rather than trying to talk yourself out of it.

Stage 6: Relapse or Termination

The ultimate goal of this phase is taking the behavior or habits you needed in order to change and taming them to the point that you no longer feel like they pose a threat. In this stage, the unhealthy habits you once had have lost their appeal. You have acquired new skills that reinforce your new lifestyle. Yet part of being human is that you're always drawn to slide back into what is automatic, familiar, and comfortable—kind of like that old bathrobe or sweatshirt sitting in the back of your closet that you quite can't force yourself to throw away. It's not unusual to relapse and creep back into old habits.

You might feel disappointed or like a failure when things seemed to be going so well and then you hit a bump in the road. One client had lost weight over several months by exercising most days and establishing a regular eating routine. Then she went on vacation with her family and ate foods she hadn't been typically eating on a regular basis, such as sugary cereals, chips, and pasta. When she returned from vacation, work demanded her attention and got it. All of it. Overwhelmed, she neglected her usual exercise routine and fell back into the pattern of work crowding out her time for self-care. To compound matters, since she wasn't exercising, she wasn't as focused on eating foods that supported her health and gave her energy. She had gotten out of the routine of allocating time to plan meals and frequenting the grocery store to stock up on healthy food supplies.

Exit Strategy: Rebounding from Relapse

The stages of change sometimes involve relapsing or falling back into old behavior. When you try to move directly into action before you're ready, you might relapse or return to your bad habits as quickly as you vowed to change. You might then beat yourself up for being so "weak" or not having any willpower. One of my clients liked to joke that she didn't just fall off the wagon, she fell off the wagon then set it on fire and pushed it off a cliff. In reality, change is a process that requires patience.

Gravitating toward familiar habits is just part of human nature, and it's good to have a sense of humor to help view the challenging times we all experience with a lighthearted and kind perspective. As my client and I worked together to regroup, she was able to step back and understand the chain of events that was causing her to relapse to old habits. We worked on identifying time in her schedule to exercise as well as to plan meals. Identifying tangible steps to take allowed her to refocus and get unstuck.

You need to shift from a mindset of change as immediate action and automatic, complete success to change as a fluid process. Keep in mind that change, like weight loss, is not a neat, perfectly straight line of progress. Though I've laid out a six-step process, the journey involves twists and turns. At some point, you might have to revert to a previous stage of change and then re-evaluate. Knowing that this is a natural part of the process frees you to focus on identifying what caused the relapse and then tweak how you want to approach it. It also lets you reconfirm your commitment to your vision and goals that sent you on your way in the first place.

CHAPTER 16

MINDFUL EATING

The problem is not in the food... The problem lies in the mind. It lies in our lack of awareness of the messages coming in from our body... Mindful eating helps us learn to hear what our body is telling us about hunger and satisfaction. It helps us become aware of who in the body/heart/mind complex is hungry, and how and what is best to nourish it.
— Jan Chozen Bays

SIMPLE IS NOT THE SAME AS EASY

So if losing weight is just a matter of eating healthier foods and smaller portions, why is losing weight and keeping it off so hard?

Because simple is not the same as easy.

Like dieting, here are some tasks that are seemingly simple but secretly complicated:

- **Folding fitted sheets.** No matter how hard I try, I end up rolling the sheets in a ball and shoving them in the cupboard.
- **Finding the opening to a plastic produce bag.** Often I stand in the produce section for what feels like five minutes, scratching at the top of the bag as I try in vain to separate the edges. Soon I begin feeling self-conscious and admiring

everyone else who has seemingly opened their bag with much less effort. If this task was an IQ test, I would fail miserably. While moistening your fingers helps, there's no way to do that without increasing risk for the spread of disease.

- **Remembering your password that you just changed.** Literally seconds after I change my password, my brain is like, *What was that again?*

- **Filling out those captcha boxes online to prove you're not a robot.** I always squint at the combination of captcha characters with puzzlement, asking myself, *Is that a capital letter? Do I put a space there?* Success usually requires at least two to three attempts to replicate the code.

- **Turning the pump of a new hand soap bottle to the open position.** First off, on a new hand soap bottle, it's really hard to see the faint imprint of the arrow and whether to turn it right or left. Often I swivel the pump handle around in endless circles, becoming increasingly frustrated as it refuses to pop up into a position where I can actually use the soap.

- **"Natural makeup"** usually requires at least five or more expensive products and 10 steps to make you look like you're not wearing anything.

- **Going to sleep when you're tired instead of staying up and watching another episode of the Netflix show you're currently into.** Your brain seductively whispers, *Just one more. You're tired already—just keeping going,* even though you know you're going to be hating yourself for that decision when the alarm hoists you out of bed in the morning.

> *My life feels like a test I didn't study for.*
> — Unknown

Diets—especially strict ones—are so popular because many of them have simple, straightforward, albeit rigid, eating rules.

When we begin a diet, we fall for the belief that limited choices and being told exactly what to eat or not eat will fix everything. Easy peasy lemon squeezy. As long as we're following the rules, we're "on track" and guaranteed quick success.

Strict diets are so appealing because in our busy and stressful lives we are happy for an opportunity where we don't have to think; we don't have to make another decision. Relieved, we can finally check our brain at the door and just be told exactly what to do. No thinking required. Weight loss then becomes another project on the to- do list with a clear beginning and end. Many of us have probably grown up with the belief that if we follow the rules, success is guaranteed. And these types of diets *are* often successful in the short term. We lose weight and think, *Yes, I've accomplished my goal.*

But then life happens.

We start to go back to our previous eating habits and feel weight begin to creep back on, or we've been so strict with our eating that deprivation chases our resolve around the corner—we start eating all our forbidden foods and can't stop—or trying to stick to the diet is consuming our life and ushering in waves of frustration and deprivation, or if we felt like we "kinda sorta" followed the diet and it didn't work, we have something else to blame: *It's the program. It's not my fault.*

We tend to resort to familiar habits because they've worn grooves in our brain that we coast along in by default. It's automatic. Sometimes when we make a change, we believe that we've "fixed" the problem and our new rules will prevent us from going back to the old ways. We start flirting with the old behavior—*I can keep cookies in the house; I'll only eat a few*—intuitively knowing we haven't reached a place yet where we can manage this kind of temptation.

Imagine that you are successful in your career and you consider yourself a high performer, yet food is the one area of life that has been a constant struggle, one that never seems to get resolved. Enter the shame spiral, in which you mistakenly beat yourself up for being so weak. You imagine that you're letting me down or that I'm going to be upset or disappointed in you, when, in reality, you are disappointed in yourself. You blame yourself, thinking that being mean to yourself or internally yelling at yourself will spur you into action. But has beating yourself up ever worked? Especially long term? Think about a time when you were yelled at for making a mistake. Did it inspire you to change, or did it cue self-loathing and make you want to hide in the bathroom and eat cookies?

Being hard on ourselves is never an effective long-term strategy. However, it's not surprising many of us fall into this belief given the messages we have heard over the years. This response is very common because it's how we've been conditioned our whole lives. Slogans have bombarded us, like "Just do it" or "Nothing tastes as good as thin feels." We have become convinced that we must suffer in order to make progress. A client who was meeting his goals was puzzled, actually, by the fact that it was easier in reality than what he thought it had to be.

Many clients come to me after trying to stick to these popular diets. In the beginning, they often experience quick, positive results, but often these results disappear just as quickly. The realization soon dawns that it's not feasible for them to continue these habits for the long term. Take, for example, a client who came to see me who was following a popular low-carb diet that restricted any type of bread, rice, pasta, or potatoes, along with most fruit. He initially lost weight but quickly grew tired of eating mostly meat and vegetables. He regained all the weight he'd lost and then some. In our discussions, to shine a light on the unsustainability of this approach, I asked, "Are you never going to eat another slice of bread ever again?"

Changing our habits and mindset that got us to this point in the first place are the keys to creating a healthy lifestyle that we can sustain for the long term.

THE MULTITASKING MYTH: HOW IT AFFECTS YOUR HEALTH

Multitasking is a badge of honor of modern life. How many times have you asked someone how they are, and they respond, "I'm so busy"? Saying we're busy or stressed is almost expected and has become a way to show our worth and prove we have value.

This might resonate with you as a caretaker. Helping others provides a form of validation and purpose. You feel compelled to "do and do" for others all the time. All this responsibility can make you feel constantly overwhelmed and fearful of ever stopping to pause or rest. You might wish you had more time for yourself, but taking care of others gives your life meaning. Without it, you might feel lost, uncertain, and uncomfortable, because you're not used to focusing on yourself. The incessant need for productivity results in paying a little bit of attention to everything at the same time that you pay attention to nothing in a substantial way. We have probably all seen videos of people walking with cell phones and then falling into fountains at the shopping mall because they're so checked out, or some similar blooper.

The same distracted mindset carries over into the way you approach eating. You feel so overwhelmed with what feels like a maxed-out brain that you give very little consideration to the food you eat. Eating becomes just another task on the list. You're in survival mode, sinking down and, as a result, you grab whatever food is available and eat it mindlessly. Years of unconscious decisions add up to weight or health that is not what you want it to be, and you think, *What happened? I didn't choose this, did I?*

MINDFULNESS: HELPING THE HELPERS

One way to change how you approach eating in a fast-paced world is by practicing mindfulness. Mindfulness is simply the moment-by-moment awareness of what's going on. It's about slowing down and tuning into the moment rather than being zoned out. It's about paying attention to what is happening in the present rather than focusing on the past or worrying about the future.

One night when I was young, my family noticed we had eaten dinner in under 10 minutes. It was a high-five type of moment; we had won a gold medal in speed eating. Yay us! Contrast that to when I visited Italy about four years ago. Meals there are served in courses consisting of appetizers; pasta, meat, or fish; salad; and dessert along with coffee and an alcoholic beverage known as a *digestivo* to help settle the stomach and digest the food. Meals last for at least two hours as the food and the conversation are savored. No Italian high fives for a fast finish.

The experience of eating slowly strengthens our ability to be present and mindful because it gives time for our body to receive the signals from our brain that we are satisfied. It helps us to start listening to cues about what and how much to eat. Mindfulness allows us to be present in the moment and connect more deeply to the food, the experience, and ultimately, ourselves.

One way I learned to practice mindfulness was experiencing the ritual of drinking Japanese green tea. Visiting Japan had always been a dream of mine, so I was thrilled when a small, Asian-inspired teahouse opened up years ago in my local area. The shop served different loose-leaf teas along with small dishes. It was my first exposure to quality loose-leaf tea, specifically Japanese green tea. The experience sparked my passion for it. I purchased some tea to make at home and learned that different types of Japanese green tea require different temperatures and amounts of water to ensure that they don't taste bitter. The ritual

of making tea makes me slow down and be in the moment by paying attention to all the details. Gyokuro is my favorite. I always
pause to sniff the intense grassy, vegetable-like scent when I open
the container. I then measure out the exact grams of tea using a
special scale, increase the water temperature just so with a tea
kettle that I can program to the exact temperature, and time the
steeping to make sure it doesn't go too long. Then I pause and
inhale the scent of tea before taking the first sip of liquid love. The
whole process inspires me to slow down and savor. It instills calm
in the busyness of the day and always leads my soul to release a
satisfied "Ahhh" after the last sip.

Three years ago, I visited Japan for the first time. I knew
I wanted to visit the country, plus I loved green tea, so I did a
search for "Japanese tea trip" on the internet. Finding a couple
who owned a small tea company in Vermont who were offering
tea tourism to Japan, I signed up and gave them my money. Four
other tourists and I visited the tea fields, where we picked the precious leaves. Then we toured the tea-processing factory, where we
watched the steaming, rolling, and drying process used to create
the finished tea. And we ended the day with a tea tasting. There
is nothing like the smell and taste of freshly processed tea. It's
sweet, fresh, grassy, and revitalizing.

Our group toured many Japanese gardens, which showcased
the mindfulness the Japanese put into everything they do. Precisely trimmed trees, beautiful flowers, fountains, small pago-
das, and old tea houses filled the outdoor spaces with peaceful
grandeur. After touring one of the garden grounds, we had the
privilege of gathering in one of the traditional old tea houses and
experiencing the formal Japanese tea ceremony for ourselves.
Every aspect of the tea ceremony held meaning, from crawling
through a low opening onto the tatami mats in the teahouse to
savoring the intricacies of making and serving a proper bowl of
matcha—powdered Japanese green tea—with the appropriate

tools and techniques. Tea is a way of life in Japan, with every aspect showing respect toward an ancient culture and tradition.

MINDFUL EATING

Slowing down and being in the moment can also be applied to the way we eat. A big part of mindfulness is about making connections. My tea trip allowed me to make a deeper connection between my drinking tea and the tea fields, processing plants, and ceremonies a world away. Mindful eating offers an alternative to strict diets; it provides a way to develop a lasting, healthy connection or partnership with your body by slowing down and giving yourself the time and grace to change your habits surrounding eating.

Eating mindfully allows us to establish a balanced eating style bite by bite. Being aware of our thoughts and then pausing to consider them gives us the time and space to decide whether or not we want to act on them. One client for whom ice cream is a trigger food convinced herself that if she started eating ice cream, she had to finish the half gallon all at once. Her internal conversation went something like this: *It's impossible for me to not eat the whole container. I have to eat it all whether or not I really want it. I have to finish it.* When we tell ourselves over and over again that something is impossible or that we have to do it, we believe the myth. It becomes so ingrained in our mind that we feel we have no choice. The ice cream becomes an evil entity forcing us to do things against our will, and we give our power away to a dessert.

Mindful.org (Mindful.org 2020), an organization dedicated to fostering mindfulness, defines the concept as "the basic human ability to be fully present, aware of where we are and what we're doing, and not overly reactive or overwhelmed by what's going on around us." To me, an important aspect of mindfulness with food is pausing, stepping back, and challenging the thoughts that tell me I have to do something or eat something and have no choice in the matter. Awareness of uncomfortable thoughts or feelings is helpful because we can remind ourselves that we don't have to obey them; we have the power to choose.

The more we exert our power, the more we believe that change is possible and the more our confidence grows to change our habits. That's why it's important to celebrate small victories. By challenging our thoughts, maybe the next time instead of eating the whole carton of ice cream or the entire sleeve of cookies, we will pause halfway through and think, *I don't need this or want this. It doesn't even taste good to me anymore. I don't have to finish this. I have a choice.* Mindful eating means tuning in, being aware, and owning our choices.

Here is another example of mindful eating. Maybe you brought some healthy snacks to work, but you're really craving a candy bar from the vending machine. You take time to consider your choices and make a conscious decision to eat the candy bar. However, instead of eating it quickly and barely tasting it, you sit at your desk, intentionally turn away from your computer, and pay attention bite by bite to how the candy looks, smells, and tastes. You rip open the wrapper and lay it on a napkin and look at the chocolate swirls on top. You then close your eyes and take a deep whiff of the chocolate with its rich cocoa smell. You take one bite and gently place the candy bar back on the napkin. Chewing slowly, you notice how the chocolate melts on your tongue as the texture changes from firm to soft and smooth. You then swallow and notice that the scent of chocolate lingers.

Why am I talking about eating a candy bar when it's possibly one of the foods you may be struggling with? Because mindful eating is not about eating only "healthy foods." It's about learning to eat food that respects your inner voice about what is pleasing to you. It's about being fully present as you eat, so your body can guide you when you feel full and satisfied. Mindful eating is about owning your choices and actively deciding to eat the candy bar instead of the apple, without judgment. You're not eating the candy bar because you're trying to fix a feeling. You're choosing to do this because you let go of judgment about what you "should" do and instead allowed your inner wisdom to guide you about what you want to do. You are never wrong when you truly listen to yourself.

Being mindful on a consistent basis is difficult for most people because of how plugged in we are as a society, but with practice, it can become as natural as breathing. Mindfulness doesn't have to be limited to eating. We can practice being aware with anything we do. While taking a walk, we can notice the colors of the sky. While removing clothes from the dryer, we can hold a fresh towel up to our nose and smell the scented detergent and feel the warmth of the cloth. While seated at the computer, we can pause and stare at a picture on the wall, noticing a new detail. Mindfulness is about being aware of the present moment and slowing down enough to tune into and cultivate an awareness of it.

Here are three steps to practice mindfulness with regard to eating:

1. Check in before Eating

Take time to become aware of the environment you're in, the food you're about to eat, and how your body feels before you start eating.

Notice your surroundings. Are you at home, at work, or in a restaurant? Are you seated or standing? Are you with other people or by yourself? Is it noisy or quiet?

Pause and look at the food on your plate. What colors and shapes are present? Stop and close your eyes and smell the food. Does it smell like you imagined?

How does your body feel? Is your stomach rumbling? Is your mouth watering? Do you feel a little light-headed because you're ready to eat or only slightly hungry?

Observe anything that slows you down and brings you into the moment.

2. Check in during Eating

The second step of mindfulness involves paying attention while you're actually eating your food. You can practice this by chewing the food slowly, paying attention to each bite. Aim to become aware of how the food tastes, including its texture, temperature, and mixture of flavors. How do these factors change as you continue to chew?

Try eating one bite of food then lowering the fork or spoon between bites. Count how many times it takes you to chew that one bite. Swallow that food and pause before taking another mouthful.

Notice how your hunger is changing. Are you starting to feel full or are you still noticing a strong desire to eat?

Hara Hachi Bu

The Japanese use the expression *hara hachi bu* (Buettner 2008, 83), or "eat until you're 80 percent full." Residents of the Japanese island of Okinawa, who are among the longest-living and healthiest people in the world, have traditionally practiced the mindfulness of hara hachi bu.

To try hara hachi bu, eat until you feel "mostly full," then wait 20 minutes. Pay attention to what the experience is like for you. Notice what 80 percent really feels like.

Stopping at 80 percent fullness is a healthy strategy because it takes the stomach time to communicate fullness to the rest of the body. Many who stop at 80 percent will feel satisfied and will ultimately eat less. If you are accustomed to eating until you are more than 80 percent full, you might find that this stopping point leaves you less sleepy and more energetic after meals.

Practicing hara hachi bu is an excellent way to play with your experience of hunger and fullness. View it as an experiment. What does it feel like to leave the table with extra room in your stomach? How difficult is it to assess that 80 percent feeling? Are there emotions or reactions that come up for you when you experiment with eating in this way? Practicing hara hachi bu helps prevent mindless eating by getting you back in touch with what it really means to go from being hungry to being satisfied.

3. Check in after Eating

When you're done eating, push your chair slightly away from the table. Sit upright in your chair with your feet on the ground and your hands on the armrest or on your lap. Center yourself, and now that you've eaten, ask yourself these questions: *How do I feel? Do I feel like I could eat more, or am I comfortably full, or stuffed beyond the gills? Is my body happy with the food choices I've made, or am I ready to lay my head down and go to sleep? Do I feel mentally satisfied? Was the food tasty, or just so-so, and I continued to eat because it was in front of me?*

Tuning in and paying attention before, during, and after eating lets you learn how to listen to your body and your mind without judgment and to balance your eating while maintaining a healthy body weight. While it takes practice, slowing down and taking time to smell, taste, and enjoy our food helps to reestablish a connection with ourselves, allowing new habits to emerge.

Mindfulness has worked wonders for my own life struggles with binge eating. Giving myself permission to eat all foods and being fully present while eating has healed my relationship with food. Recently, I made a homemade pizza that at an earlier time in my life would have been tempted me to devour it all at once. This time, however, I approached the whole experience in a way that was very satisfying for me, so I felt no need to overwhelm myself with large portions. I chose a nice, crispy crust along with five different kinds of shredded cheese and my favorite pizza sauce. Before I started eating, I looked at the toasted marks from the pizza stone on bottom of the crust, noticing how the cheese had melted from fine shreds into a pool of gooeyness. Taking a bite, I heard the crunch of the crust and tasted the freshness of the sautéed green peppers against the sweetness of the pizza sauce. After dinner I wanted something sweet. Without judgment, I asked myself what I was craving. My rational brain might have argued for a piece of fruit or told me to skip dessert altogether since I had eaten pizza, but my intuitive brain knew I really wanted some ice cream. So I took out a small dish, dished up a scoop, and ate it slowly, without other distractions, savoring the creaminess of the ice cream as it started to melt a little. Once I finished that, I still wanted a little more, so I dished out another small scoop and savored every bite. I felt very satisfied because I ate at a pace that I could be in the moment and mindful of what I was eating.

Allowing myself to eat what I wanted without judgment supported eating a portion that was just the right amount for my hunger. Giving myself permission to eat these foods has freed me from the feeling of deprivation that used to drive me to eat as much as I could before forbidding myself from ever eating them again. Honoring our hunger is one way we honor and ultimately heal ourselves.

CHAPTER 17

SMALL STEPS TO A BIG LIFE

You don't have to see the whole staircase,
just take the first step.
— Martin Luther King, Jr.

Years ago, I couldn't understand why people would choose to run for exercise. At the time, I enjoyed taking dance aerobics classes and walking but couldn't comprehend the appeal of this activity. I would see people running in my neighborhood while I was driving to carry out errands and all I could think was, *Why would you choose to do that?* Running seemed so difficult and the thought of deriving any kind of enjoyment from it mind-boggled me.

At the same time, I was planning to do some travel, and the practical side of me knew that running would be an efficient way to get an intense workout in without having to find a gym. I knew I was limiting myself by not exploring running as a possible workout option, so I made a decision that I was going to get over my personal bias hump and at least try it.

I started by alternating walking one block and then jogging the next. A block seemed like a digestible distance, and my mind told me, *I can do that.* Little by little, I increased the distance— walking one block and jogging two blocks. I will never forget the day I jogged for 15 minutes straight. It was a beautiful Saturday morning, the kind of day I like to call San Diego weather—moderately warm in the 70s with a clear, blue sky that just makes a person feel good to be outside. I was so excited because I was scheduled to bring home my eight-week-old puppy, Barkley, a black Lab/bullmastiff mix—a new companion for my dog, Tilly. The swirling energy and joy around picking up Barkley sent me floating down the street. Not until I stopped and glanced at my watch did I see that I had run for 15 minutes continuously. Floored, I did a double take! This was a major victory for me since I didn't think I would ever be able to do such a thing. The high from accomplishing this new feat opened the door to possibility. Something I had originally closed myself off to was now an option. My world had just gotten a little bit bigger. This story is an example of how we can do the "hard stuff" and accomplish big things when we break it down into smaller pieces.

FIRST STEP: CHALLENGING OUR ASSUMPTIONS

How often have you limited yourself by making the decision beforehand that you can't do something or told yourself it's not possible? Or that if you aren't able to do something perfectly, you give up rather than get started? Or that the goal feels so overwhelming you already feel defeated and become unable to take action?

I never thought I would ever be a runner, but years later, I've completed many races and am now training for my third marathon. I'm a self-admitted, solidly upper-average, plodding-along runner. I'm not slow or particularly fast or very graceful, but it doesn't matter. The joy that fills me from being outside enjoying the fresh air and the freedom of movement is what matters to me. If I had never challenged my assumptions and at least tried running out, I never would have discovered a new, enjoyable way to move that supports my physical and mental well-being.

You never know what you're capable of doing until you try. Challenging your assumptions about what you can and can't do is the first step to change. The next step is to take your larger task or goal and break it into smaller pieces to help spark action. When I learned how to run, I started small and built up from there. For instance, if you want to complete a marathon but have never run before, do you go out and try to jog five miles on the first day? Of course not. The same holds true for personal "marathons" or "ultramarathons." If you try to change everything at once, you're likely to become quickly overwhelmed and quit.

> *If you think you are too small to make a difference, try*
> *sleeping with a mosquito.*
> — Dalai Lama

You might think that small changes are insignificant, but, like a mosquito, they definitely can have a big impact. Underestimating the value of consistent small changes keeps you stuck because it fosters the all-or-nothing or "light-switch" mentality I addressed earlier. You feel that unless you can make swift and epic changes perfectly, they are not worth doing. You become paralyzed from taking any action, which then fosters the cycle of feeling over-whelmed and discouraged. Small changes or commitments have a bigger meaning than just changing your behavior. Daily small steps are the promises you make to yourself. They are the ultimate act of self-love as they confirm that you matter, and you are important. It reminds you that you deserve the self-care you give to others.

SECOND STEP: BEING AWARE OF THE MOTIVATION MYTH

> *Some mornings you wake up needing*
> *a cup of coffee and a million dollars.*
> — Anonymous

People often beat themselves up because they assume that everyone else is motivated and that there must be something wrong with them, but this is not the case. Motivation is like that million dollars. It would be great to have, and it definitely makes life easier, but it's generally not something you can rely on or expect to magically be present. Relying on motivation is like trying to build your foundation on quicksand. Some days you may have it, and everything may seem OK. But the ground can shift beneath you. Entire industries are devoted to motivational posters, calendars, coffee mugs, and t-shirts. I like an inspirational quote as much as the next person, but the idea that you're always going to feel motivated is a myth. There is a difference between being interested and committed. When you are interested, you do something when it's easy. When you are committed, you do it no matter what. As we talked about in Chapter 6, this is the reason it's so important to be tied into your "why" to help you keep going on difficult days. Motivation is never guaranteed.

Cupcakes are muffins that believed in miracles.
— Anonymous

If motivation isn't enough, how can we tackle the hard stuff, including changing our relationship with food? Like constructing a house, you want to start building a strong foundation with consistent habits. The key is to start with small, daily actions and work on expanding them.

SOLUTION ONE: THE 10-MINUTE RULE

We build our character from the bricks
of habit we pile up day by day.
— Zig Ziglar

How do you take action if you feel like every fiber in your being is fighting against you? It's important to remember that moods and emotions are temporary. While you want to listen to yourself, you also must be aware that internal dialogue can be deceptive and weave a story that may not be accurate. For example, I exercise daily, but do I always feel inspired to do so? Nope! You should hear the internal conversation on most days: *I'm tired. I'm stressed. I think I'm working too hard. Maybe I need to take a day off.* Everyone has to find their own balance, but I've worked out long enough to know myself and that once I get started, I'm fine and feel so much better afterward.

I give myself the 10-minute rule. If I absolutely can't continue exercising after 10 minutes, I allow myself to take a day off. But guess what? After 10 minutes, I start to think, *Eh, this isn't so bad.* Accomplishing a goal in smaller increments can help reduce mental hurdles. *If I could do 10 minutes, what's 10 more minutes? I can do anything for 10 minutes. After that, I can stop if I want to.* But I usually keep going because I know I can continue. By then, I'm into it and happy I didn't give myself a total "out." I also keep going because this is a self-care promise I made to myself. Exercise allows me to be in the moment and do something that is just for me. It's one of the ways I honor myself and remind myself I deserve to be taken care of, too.

SOLUTION TWO: BE PART OF THE 1 PERCENT

The 10-minute rule I created for myself is reflective of a bigger philosophy called the Kaizen effect (Kaizen 2020), which focuses on small, continual improvement. This philosophy was originally developed by American business management theorists during World War II to help businesses look for incremental ways to make improvements on existing jobs with the resources they had.

Americans then introduced this concept to Japanese factories after World War II to help them rebuild their economy. The Japanese named it Kaizen, and it blossomed into a larger business philosophy of continuous improvement.

Kaizen can be applied to your health journey as well. Instead of looking for the magic answer that will instantly make everything better, focus on trying to be 1 percent better each day. If you want to move more, aim to walk for five minutes each day and then increase from there. Want to change your eating habits? Eat one piece of fruit each day. Small, consistent changes may not seem to have a big effect as you start, but your investment compounds and builds each day. Gradually you will notice things are shifting and gaining momentum. Be focused on your destination but embrace the process to get there. Steps—no matter how small—still move you in the direction you want to go.

CHAPTER 18

GRAVITY

Challenges are gifts that force us to search
for a new center of gravity. Don't fight them.
Just find a new way to stand.
— Oprah Winfrey

I will never forget standing in the middle of my living room in an empty, ground-floor apartment, staring out the back patio door at the green grass and trees. The movers had just deposited the last of my boxes, leaving me alone in the silence trying to process the moment. I was in the midst of a divorce after 17 years of marriage, and this was my first place after moving out of my house. My mind traveled back to the poster that my childhood self studied years ago on our basement wall of the tiny duckling waddling into the world. The same nervous, overwhelmed, scared-but-also-excited feelings arose in me at that moment as I faced the possibilities of new beginnings. I searched for my new center of gravity, reassuring myself with what would become a daily mantra: *I'm OK. I'll figure this out.*

After taking the journey through this book with me, you might now be feeling like I felt in that moment—nervous and a bit overwhelmed about making changes but excited about the possibilities and more confident about your ability to start moving forward. The purpose of this book was to help you look at how you approach food and to realize that the issues you struggle with are not about the food itself but about deeper emotions rooted in the past and present. They are about how you see yourself both now and in the future. The influence of your mindset as you move forward cannot be overstated.

My goal has been to provide techniques and strategies to help you start creating your own toolbox, to not only change habits but also retrain your brain to acknowledge and handle emotions, practice mindfulness, and, most importantly, reinvigorate your belief in yourself. I want you to know that you can be successful no matter where you are now and no matter what has happened in the past. Be reassured that to change your life, you don't have to change everything at once. Just choosing one thing—such as acknowledging an emotion, pausing for a moment before eating, or deciding to add some movement to your life—are all steps in the right direction. Daily practice of these habits will allow you to slowly build on the foundation you are creating and gain momentum over time. Consistent action will nourish your strong roots, allowing you to fully stand in your power.

Remember to celebrate your victories each time you make a different choice that honors yourself. You deserve to be loved and taken care of as well as you take care of others.

My hope is that I have helped you to start finding a new center of gravity and a new way to stand. I have shared my story with you to let you know there is hope. I'm living proof of that. If you're feeling like that small duckling from my childhood poster, know that the little duckling is no longer alone. My wish is that this book has given you the sense and reassurance that I'm standing right there beside you, saying, "You and your story matter. You are not alone. We'll figure this out together."

WORKS CITED

Buettner, Dan. 2010. *The Blue Zones: Lessons for Living Longer from the People Who've Lived the Longest*. Washington, DC: National Geographic Society.

Burton, Susan. 2020. *Empty: A Memoir*. New York: Random House.

Caliper. *Making it in the "Bigs" How Mental Toughness Differentiates NCAA Division I and Professional Athletes*. Princeton: Caliper, 2020.

Coker Ross, Carolyn. 2017. Review of *What You Need to Know to Get Better: Getting to the Root Cause To Treat Eating Disorders*. 2017. https://www.nationaleatingdisorders.org/blog/eating-disorders-trauma-ptsd-recovery.

Danowski, Debbie. 2006. *The Emotional Eater's Book of Inspiration: 90 Truths You Need to Know to Overcome Your Food Addiction*. New York: Da Capo Lifelong Books.

Fangyuan Chen, Rocky Peng Chen, Li Yang. 2019. "When Sadness Comes Alive, Will It Be Less Painful? The Effects of Anthropomorphic Thinking on Sadness Regulation and Consumption." *Journal of Consumer Psychology* 30 (2): 277–95. https://doi.org/10.1002/jcpy.1137.

Gilbert, Elizabeth. 2017. *Eat, Pray, Love: One Woman's Search for Everything Across Italy, India and Indonesia*. New York: Riverhead Books.

Grohol, John. 2019. "15 Common Cognitive Distortions." Psych Central. January 17, 2019. https://psychcentral.com/lib/15-common-cognitive-distortions/.

Huget, Jennifer LaRue. 2010. "The Downside of Downsizing." *Washingtonpost.com*. December 7. https://www.washingtonpost.com/wp-dyn/content/article/2010/12/07/AR2010120702271.html.

n.d. Review of "*Kaizen | Kaizen Methodology | Quality-One*." Accessed 2020. https://quality-one.com/kaizen/.

LeVan, Angie. 2009. Review of *Seeing Is Believing: The Power of Visualization. Psychology Today, 2009.* https://www.psychologytoday.com/us/blog/flourish/200912/seeing-is-believing-the-power-visualization.

Mindful Staff. 2019. "What Is Mindfulness?" Mindful. January 8, 2020. Accessed December 29, 2020. https://www.mindful.org/what-is-mindfulness/.

Snetselaar, Linda G. n.d. Review of *Counseling for Change*. In *Krause's Food, Nutrition, & Diet Therapy, 11th Edition*, 520–21. Philadelphia: Elsevier.

2012. Review of *Brief Cognitive–Behavioral Therapy. In Brief Interventions and Brief Therapies for Substance Abuse: Treatment Improvement Protocol Series 34*, 63. Rockville: U.S. Department of Health and Human Services.

Walsh, Peter. 2009. *Does This Clutter Make My Butt Look Fat?* London: Simon & Schuster.

Warner, Jennifer. n.d. "People Pleasers May Overeat at Parties." WebMD. https://www.webmd.com/diet/news/20120203/people-pleasers-may-overeat-at-parties#1.

Yin, Henry H., and Barbara J. Knowlton. 2006. "The Role of the Basal Ganglia in Habit Formation." *Nature Reviews Neuroscience* 7 (6): 464–476. https://doi.org/10.1038/nrn1919.

QUOTE RESOURCES

Alexandra Elle. Good Reads.com, Good Reads LLC, 2020. https://www.goodreads.com/quotes/1177779-i-am-thankful-for-my-struggle-because-without-it-i, accessed December 29, 2020.

Aristotle. AZQuotes.com, Wind and Fly LTD, 2020. https://www.azquotes.com/quote/1413247, accessed December 29, 2020.

Bear Grylls. AZQuotes.com, Wind and Fly LTD, 2020. https://www.azquotes.com/quote/118613, accessed December 29, 2020.

Dalai Lama. AZQuotes.com, Wind and Fly LTD, 2020. https://www.azquotes.com/quote/345708, accessed December 29, 2020.

Deepak Chopra. AZQuotes.com, Wind and Fly LTD, 2020. https://www.azquotes.com/quote/1445036, accessed December 29, 2020.

Dodinsky. Good Reads.com, Good Reads LLC, 2020. https://www.goodreads.com/author/quotes/6508916.Dodinsky, accessed December 29, 2020.

Edmund Lee. Good Reads.com, Good Reads LLC, 2020. https://www.goodreads.com/quotes/813062-surround-yourself-with-the-dreamers-and-the-doers-the-believers, accessed December 29, 2020.

Elisabeth Kubler-Ross. AZQuotes.com, Wind and Fly LTD, 2020. https://www.azquotes.com/quote/163916, accessed December 29, 2020.

Elizabeth Gilbert. AZQuotes.com, Wind and Fly LTD, 2020. https://www.azquotes.com/quote/401700, accessed December 29, 2020.

Friedrich Nietzsche. AZQuotes.com, Wind and Fly LTD, 2020. https://www.azquotes.com/quote/214473, accessed December 29, 2020.

Giada De Laurentiis. AZQuotes.com, Wind and Fly LTD, 2020. https://www.azquotes.com/quote/84692, accessed December 29, 2020.

Jan Chozen Bays. AZQuotes.com, Wind and Fly LTD, 2020. https://www.azquotes.com/quote/945760, accessed December 29, 2020.

Ken Wheaton. Good Reads.com, Good Reads LLC, 2020. https://www.goodreads.com/work/quotes/26411414-sweet-as-cane-salty-as-tears, accessed December 29, 2020.

Iyanla Vanzant. AZQuotes.com, Wind and Fly LTD, 2020. https://www.azquotes.com/quote/727926, accessed December 29, 2020.

Lao Tzu. Good Reads.com, Good Reads LLC, 2020. https://www.goodreads.com/quotes/21535-the-journey-of-a-thousand-miles-begins-with-a-single, accessed December 29, 2020.

Mandy Hale. Good Reads.com, Good Reads LLC, 2020. https://www.goodreads.com/quotes/1023321-growth-is-painful-change-is-painful-but-nothing-is-as, accessed December 29, 2020.

Martin Luther King, Jr. AZQuotes.com, Wind and Fly LTD, 2020. https://www.azquotes.com/quote/543445, accessed December 29, 2020.

Michael Jordan. AZQuotes.com, Wind and Fly LTD, 2020. https://www.azquotes.com/quote/393622, accessed December 29, 2020.

Oprah Winfrey. AZQuotes.com, Wind and Fly LTD, 202. https://www.azquotes.com/quote/355851 accessed December 29, 2020.

Paulo Coelho. AZQuotes.com, Wind and Fly LTD, 2020. https://www.azquotes.com/quote/591295, accessed December 29, 2020.

Ralph Waldo Emerson. AZQuotes.com, Wind and Fly LTD, 2020. https://www.azquotes.com/quote/591015, accessed December 29, 2020.

Randy Pausch. AZQuotes.com, Wind and Fly LTD, 2020. https://www.azquotes.com/quote/356771, accessed December 29, 2020.

Roy T. Bennett. Good Reads.com, Good Reads LLC, 2020. https://www.goodreads.com/quotes/8014046-the-biggest-wall-you-have-to-climb-is-the-one, accessed December 29, 2020.

Zig Ziglar. AZQuotes.com, Wind and Fly LTD, 2020. https://www.azquotes.com/quote/892432, accessed December 29, 2020.

ABOUT THE AUTHOR

Mary Perry is a Registered Dietitian with a passion for health and fitness and a strong desire to help others build a healthy relationship with food.

Mary had a successful professional career in the federal government but struggled with her weight since childhood, alternating between bouts of restrictive eating and binge-ing. After overcoming her own food issues, she returned to school to build professional expertise in order to help others.

In her dietetic career, Mary has worked with thousands of people in private practice, medical offices, corporate wellness programs, and health clubs. Whether you are starting your journey to change, or have been struggling for years, Mary tailors her counseling to help you achieve a new mindset.

Mary graduated from James Madison University with a bachelor of science in dietetics. She also has a bachelor of arts in political science and a master's degree in public administration.

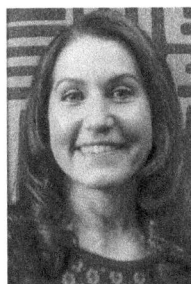

www.ingramcontent.com/pod-product-compliance
Lightning Source LLC
Chambersburg PA
CBHW050841270326
41930CB00019B/3429